TEACHINGS OF SWAMI VIVEKANANDA

TEACHINGS OF SWAMI VIVEKANANDA

*"The older I grow, the more everything
seems to me to lie in manliness.
This is my new gospel."*

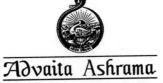

Advaita Ashrama
(PUBLICATION DEPARTMENT)
5 DEHI ENTALLY ROAD · KOLKATA 700 014

Published by
Swami Bodhasarananda
Adhyaksha, Advaita Ashrama
Mayavati, Champawat, Uttarakhand, Himalayas
from its Publication Department, Kolkata
Email: mail@advaitaashrama.org
Website: www.advaitaashrama.org

© *All Rights Reserved*
Twenty-eighth Reprint, August 2013
3M3C

ISBN 978-81-85301-87-7

Printed in India at
Trio Process
Kolkata 700 014

PREFACE TO THE FIRST EDITION

It is an undoubted fact that the message of Swami Vivekananda has influenced, inspired, and transformed hundreds of lives. Here in the following pages are given some quotations from the great Swami for the benefit of those who have not read him or who cannot make time to go through his voluminous writings and speeches, so that they may get at least a partial glimpse of the strength and sublimity of his teachings. These quotations may be helpful even to those who have studied his works. For sometimes one or two words of this great dynamic personality are sufficient to invigorate a drooping spirit, or to awaken one to a new sense of hope and courage when everything seems dark and circumstances appear insurmountable. When one reads the writings of a person like Swami Vivekananda who has touched on so many topics of our individual and national life, one is sure to have one's own choice of his sayings or preference for particular passages. It is but natural. So any selection, however careful, will be found incomplete. The compiler will consider his labour fruitful, if the following selections will create in one a desire to read Swami Vivekananda more thoroughly and find out for oneself what phase of his message appeals to him most.

ADVAITA ASHRAMA
MAYAVATI, HIMALAYAS
February 1, 1948

PREFACE TO THE SECOND EDITION

This edition has been carefully revised and also enlarged. Sections XI, XXX, and XLIII have been added.[1]

February 15, 1953

PREFACE TO THE FOURTH EDITION

In this edition the book is further revised and enlarged by adding section XXXVII on Ramakrishna, as also a few passages under the existing sections. We have also included a biographical introduction by Christopher Isherwood, published in *What Religion Is*, with the kind permission of Messrs J. M. Dent and Sons Ltd., London, and of the Julian Press Inc., New York. We hope it will be read with interest.

The references at the end of each passage are

---

[1] Sections XXX and XLIII are renumbered XXXI and XXXII respectively in the present edition.

to the latest editions of *The Complete Works of Swami Vivekananda.*

February 18, 1964

PREFACE TO THE FIFTH EDITION

In this edition four passages have been added, one each to sections V, XXV, XXVII, and XXXVIII, bringing the total number to one thousand.

The references at the end of the passages have been corrected according to the latest editions of the various volumes of *The Complete Works of Swami Vivekananda* as follows: I—13th ed., 1970; II—11th ed., 1968; III—10th ed., 1970; IV—9th ed., 1966; V—9th ed., 1970; VI—8th ed., 1968; VII—7th ed., 1969; VIII—4th ed., 1964.

June 16, 1971   PUBLISHER

CONTENTS

		PAGE
	PREFACE	iii
	INTRODUCTION	ix
I	ATMAN OR THE SELF	1
II	BHAKTI OR THE LOVE OF GOD	7
III	BRAHMAN OR THE SUPREME REALITY	19
IV	BUDDHA	23
V	BUDDHISM	29
VI	CHRIST	33
VII	CHRISTIANITY	38
VIII	CONCENTRATION	41
IX	DUTY	45
X	EDUCATION	50
XI	ETHICS	56
XII	FAITH	63
XIII	FOOD	68
XIV	FREEDOM AND MUKTI (SALVATION)	73
XV	GITA	82
XVI	GOD	88
XVII	GURU OR THE SPIRITUAL GUIDE	99
XVIII	HAPPINESS	103
XIX	HINDUISM	109
XX	HINDUS	115

		PAGE
XXI	THE HOUSEHOLDER'S LIFE	119
XXII	IDEAL WOMANHOOD	124
XXIII	IMAGE WORSHIP	138
XXIV	INCARNATION	145
XXV	INDIA—CAUSE OF HER DEGENERATION	150
XXVI	INDIA—HER CHARACTERISTICS	156
XXVII	INDIA—THE WAY TO HER REGENERATION	161
XXVIII	KRISHNA AND KARMA-YOGA	173
XXIX	KNOWLEDGE AND IGNORANCE	186
XXX	MAN	192
XXXI	MAYA	198
XXXII	MEDITATION	205
XXXIII	MIND AND THOUGHT	210
XXXIV	MOHAMMED AND ISLAM	214
XXXV	NON-INJURY	219
XXXVI	ONENESS	223
XXXVII	RAMAKRISHNA	226
XXXVIII	RELIGION	237
XXXIX	SANNYASA OR THE MONASTIC LIFE	248
XL	SERVICE	258
XLI	STRENGTH	263
XLII	UPANISHADS	269
XLIII	VEDANTA: ITS THEORY & PRACTICE	276
XLIV	YOGA	293

INTRODUCTION

One morning early in September 1893, a lady named Mrs. George W. Hale looked out through a window of her handsome home on Chicago's Dearborn Avenue and saw, seated on the opposite side of the street, a young man of Oriental appearance who was dressed in a turban and the ochre robe of a Hindu monk.

Mrs. Hale was, fortunately, not a conventional woman. She did not call the police to tell the stranger to move on; she did not even ring for the servants to go and ask him what he wanted. She noticed that he was unshaven and that his clothes were crumpled and dirty, but she was aware, also, that there was a kind of royal air about him. There he sat, perfectly composed, meditative, serene. He did not look as if he had lost his way. (And, indeed, he was quite the opposite of lost, for he had just resigned himself to the will of God.) Mrs. Hale suddenly made a most intelligent guess; coming out of her house and crossing the street, she asked him politely, "Sir, are you a delegate to the Parliament of Religions?"

She was answered with equal politeness, in fluent educated English. The stranger introduced himself as Swami Vivekananda and told her that he had indeed come to Chicago to attend the meetings of the Parliament, although he was not officially a delegate. As a matter of fact, he had first arrived in Chicago from India in the middle of July, only to find that the Parliament's opening had been postponed till September. His money was running short and someone had advised him that he would be able to live more cheaply in Boston, so he had taken the train there. On the train, he had met a lady who had invited him to stay at her home, which was called "Breezy Meadows". Since then, he had given talks to various church and social groups, been asked a lot of silly questions about his country, been laughed at by children because of his funny clothes. The day before yesterday, Professor J. H. Wright, who taught Greek at Harvard University, had bought him a ticket back to Chicago, assuring him that he would be welcome at the Parliament, even though he had no invitation: "To ask you, Swami, for credentials is like asking the sun if it has permission to shine." The Professor had also given him the address of the committee which was in charge of the delegates to the Parliament, but this address Vivekananda somehow lost on his way to Chicago. He tried to get information from passers-by on the street but, as ill luck would have it, the station was situated in the midst of a district where German was chiefly spoken, and the Swami could not make himself understood. Meanwhile, night was coming on. The Swami did not know how to obtain or use a city directory and so was at a loss how to find a suitable hotel. It seemed to him simpler to sleep in a big empty boxcar in the freight yards of the railroad. Next morning, hungry and rumpled, he woke, as he put it, "smelling fresh water", and had begun to walk in a direction which brought him, sure enough, to the edge of Lake Michigan. But the wealthy homes of Lake Shore Drive proved inhospitable; he had knocked at the doors of several and had been rudely turned away. At length, after further wanderings, he had found himself here, and had decided to go no further but to sit down and await whatever event God might send. And now, Vivekananda concluded, "What a romantic deliverance! How strange are the ways of the Lord!"

Mrs. Hale must have laughed as she listened to this; for Vivekananda always related his adventures and misadventures with humour, and his own deep chuckles were most infectious. They went back together into the house, where the Swami was invited to wash and shave and eat breakfast. Mrs. Hale then accompanied him to the headquarters of the committee, which arranged for his accommodation with the other Oriental delegates to the Parliament.

The idea of holding a Parliament of Religions in Chicago had been conceived at least five years before this, in relation to the main project of the World's Columbian Exposition, which was to be held to commemorate the four-hundredth anniversary of the discovery of America by Columbus. The Exposition was designed to demonstrate Western Man's material progress, especially in science and technology. It was agreed, however, that all forms of progress must be represented, and there were congresses devoted to such varied themes as woman's progress, the public press, medicine and surgery, temperance, commerce and finance, music, government and legal reform, economic science, and—strange as it may sound to us nowadays—Sunday rest. And since, to quote the official language of the committee, "faith in a Divine Power has been, like the sun, a light-giving and fructifying potency in Man's intellectual and moral development", there had also to be a Parliament of Religions.

One may smile at all the pomposity, but it must be agreed that the calling of such a parliament was a historic act of liberalism. This was probably the first time in the history of the world that representatives of all the major religions had been brought together in one place, with freedom to express their beliefs. Paradoxically, the most genuinely liberal of the Parliament's organisers were the agnostics; for they were interested solely in promoting inter-religious tolerance. The zealous Christians took a less impartial view, as was only to be expected. In the words of a Catholic priest: "It is not true that all religions are equally good; but neither is it true that all religions except one are no good at all. The Christianity of the future, more just than that of the past, will assign to each its place in that work of evangelical preparation which the elder doctors of the Church discern in heathenism itself, and which is not yet completed." In other words, heathenism has its uses as a preparation for Christianity.

But what really mattered was the acceptance of an invitation to preside at the Parliament by Cardinal Gibbons, leader of the American Catholics. This was all the more valuable because the Archbishop of Canterbury had refused to attend, objecting that the very meeting of such a parliament implied the equality of all religions. In addition to the Christians, the Buddhists, the Hindus, the Moslems, the Jews, the Confucianists, the Shintoists, the Zoroastrians, and a number of smaller sects and groups were represented. Vivekananda could, of course, be counted as a recruit to the Hindu delegation; but in fact, as we shall see, he was standing for something larger than any one sect; the ancient Indian doctrine of the universality of spiritual truth.

When the Parliament opened, on the morning of 11th September, Vivekananda immediately attracted notice as one of the most striking figures seated on the platform, with his splendid robe, yellow turban, and handsome bronze face. In his photographs, one is struck by the largeness of his features—they have something of the lion about them—the broad strong nose, the full expressive lips, the great dark burning eyes. Eye-witnesses were also impressed by the majesty of his presence. Though powerfully built, Vivekananda was about medium height, but he seems always to have created the effect of bigness. It was said of him that, despite his size, he moved with a natural masculine grace; "like a great cat", as one lady expressed it. In America, he was frequently taken for an Indian prince or aristocrat, because of his quiet but assured air of command.

Others commented on his look of being "inly-pleased"; he seemed able to draw upon inner reserves of strength at all times, and there was a humorous, watchful gleam in his eyes which suggested calm, amused detachment of spirit. Everyone responded to the extraordinarily deep, bell-like beauty of his voice; certain of its vibrations caused a mysterious psychic excitement among his hearers. And no doubt this had something to do with the astonishing reaction of the audience to Vivekananda's first speech.

During that first morning's session, Vivekananda's turn came to speak; but he excused himself and asked for more time. Later, in a letter to friends in India, he confessed that he had been suffering from stage fright. All the other delegates had prepared addresses; he had none. However, this hesitation only increased the general interest in him.

At length, during the afternoon, Vivekananda rose to his feet. In his deep voice, he began, "Sisters and Brothers of America"—and the entire audience, many hundred people, clapped and cheered wildly for two whole minutes. Hitherto, the audience had certainly been well-disposed; some of the speakers had been greeted enthusiastically and all of them with sufficient politeness. But nothing like this demonstration had taken place. No doubt the vast majority of those present hardly knew why they had been so powerfully moved. The appearance, even the voice, of Vivekananda cannot fully explain it. A large gathering has its own strange kind of subconscious telepathy, and this one must have been somehow aware that it was in the presence of that most unusual of all beings, a man whose words express exactly what he is. When Vivekananda said, "Sisters and Brothers", he actually meant that he regarded the American women and men before him as his sisters and brothers: the well-worn oratorical phrase became simple truth.

As soon as they would let him, the Swami continued his speech. It was quite a short one, pleading for universal tolerance and stressing the common basis of all religions. When it was over, there was more, thunderous applause. A lady who was present recalled later, "I saw scores of women walking over the benches to get near him, and I said to myself, 'Well, my lad, if you can resist that onslaught you are indeed a God!'" Such onslaughts were to become a part of the daily discipline of Vivekananda's life in America.

He made several more speeches during the days that followed, including an important statement of the nature and ideals of Hinduism. By the time the Parliament had come to an end, he was, beyond comparison, its most popular speaker. He had his pick of social invitations. A lecture bureau offered to organise a tour for him; and he accepted.

In those days, when the Frontier was still a living memory, one did not have to go far from the great cities to find oneself in the pioneer world of the tent-show. Politicians, philosophers, writers, the great Sarah Bernhardt herself—all were treated more or less as circus attractions. Even today, the name "Swami" is associated with theatrical trickery, and most Americans are quite unaware that those who have the right to call themselves by it have taken formal monastic vows; that it is, in fact, a title just as worthy of respect as that of "Father" in the Catholic Church. Vivekananda called himself Swami, and therefore, in the eyes of the public, he was regarded as some kind of an entertainer; he might hope for applause but he could expect no consideration for his privacy. He had to face the crudest publicity, the most brutal curiosity, hospitality which was lavish but ruthless and utterly exhausting. It exhausted him and eventually wrecked his health but, for the time being, he was equal to it and even seemed to enjoy it. He was outspoken to the point of bluntness, never at a loss for repartee, never thrown off balance even when he roared with momentary indignation because of some idiotic question about his "heathen" countrymen. No one could laugh at him as he laughed at himself; for no one else could appreciate the rich and subtle joke of his very presence in these surroundings—a monk preaching in a circus!

Vivekananda had come to America to speak for his native land. He wanted to tell Americans about India's poverty and appeal for their help.

But he also had a message to the West. He asked his hearers to forsake their materialism and learn from the ancient spirituality of the Hindus. What he was working for was an exchange of values. He recognised great virtues in the West—energy and initiative and courage—which he found lacking among Indians; and he had not come to America in a spirit of negative criticism. It is significant that when, during the earliest days of his visit, he was taken to see a prison near Boston, his reaction was as follows:

> How benevolently the inmates are treated, how they are reformed and sent back as useful members of society—how grand, how beautiful, you must see to believe! And oh, how my heart ached to think of what we think of the poor, the low, in India. They have no chance, no escape, no way to climb up. They sink lower and lower every day.

Yet he offended many by his outspokenness, "In New York", he used to say smilingly, "I have emptied entire halls." And no wonder! To the ears of rigid fundamentalists, his teaching of Man's essential divinity must have sounded utterly blasphemous, especially as it was presented in his picturesque, serio-comic phrases: "Look at the ocean and not at the wave; see no difference between ant and angel. Every worm is the brother of the Nazarene.... Obey the scriptures until you are strong enough to do without them.... Every man in Christian countries has a huge cathedral on his head, and on top of that a book.... The range of idols is from wood and stone to Jesus and Buddha...." Vivekananda taught that God is within each one of us, and that each one of us was born to rediscover his own God-nature. His favourite story was of a lion who imagined himself to be a sheep, until another lion showed him his reflection in a pool. "And you are lions", he would tell his hearers, "you are pure, infinite, and perfect souls.... He, for whom you have been weeping and praying in churches and temples ... is your own Self." He was the prophet of self-reliance, of individual search and effort.

He spoke little about the cults of Hinduism—the particular devotion to Rama, Kali, Vishnu, or Krishna which is practised by the devotees of the various sects. It was only occasionally that Vivekananda referred to his own personal cult and revealed that he, too, had a Master whom he regarded as a divine incarnation—a Master named Ramakrishna, who had died less than ten years previously, and whom he himself had intimately known.

Vivekananda was a very great devotee; but he did not proclaim his devotion to all comers. His refusal to do so was a considered decision.

Speaking of his work in America after returning to India, he said: "If I had preached the personality of Ramakrishna, I might have converted half the world; but that kind of conversion is short-lived. So instead I preached Ramakrishna's principles. If people accept the principles, they will eventually accept the personality."

At the time of the Parliament of Religions, Vivekananda was only thirty years old; he had been born in Calcutta on 12th January 1863. The name of his family was Datta, and his parents gave him the name Narendranath; Naren for short. As a monk, he had wandered about India under various names; he assumed the name of Vivekananda only just before embarking for the United States, at the suggestion of the Maharaja of Khetri, who, with the Maharaja of Mysore, paid the expenses of his journey. Viveka is a Sanskrit word meaning discrimination, more particularly in the philosophic sense of discrimination between the real (God) and the unreal (the phenomena recognised by our sense-perceptions). Ananda means divine bliss, or the peace which is obtained through enlightenment; it is a frequently used suffix to any name which is assumed by a monk.

When Naren was in his middle teens, he started going to college in Calcutta. He was a good-looking, athletic youth and extremely intelligent. He was also a fine singer and could play several musical instruments. Already, he showed a great power for leadership among the boys of his own age. His teachers felt sure that he was destined to make a mark in life.

At that period, Calcutta was the chief port of entry for European ideas and cultural influences; and no young Indian student could remain unaffected by them. To meet the challenge of missionary Christianity, a movement had been formed to modernise Hinduism—to do away with ancient ritual and priestcraft, to emancipate women, and to abolish child marriage. This movement was called the Brahmo Samaj. Naren joined it, but soon found its aims superficial; they did not satisfy his own spiritual needs. He read Hume, Herbert Spencer, and John Stuart Mill, and began to call himself an agnostic. His parents urged him to marry, but he refused, feeling that he must remain chaste and unattached so as to be ready to devote himself body and soul to a great cause. What cause? He did not yet exactly know. He was still looking for someone and something in which he could whole-heartedly believe. Meanwhile, his restless and fearless spirit was on fire for action.

It so happened that a relative of Naren's was a devotee of Ramakrishna, and that one of Naren's teachers, Professor Hastie, was among the few Englishmen who had ever met him. What these two had to say about Ramakrishna excited Naren's curiosity. Then, in November 1881, he was invited to sing at a house where Ramakrishna was a guest. They had a brief conversation and Ramakrishna invited the young man to come and visit him at the Dakshineswar Temple, on the Ganga a few miles outside Calcutta, where he lived.

From the first, Naren was intrigued and puzzled by Ramakrishna's personality. He had never met anyone quite like this slender, bearded man in his middle forties who had the innocent directness of a child. He had about him an air of intense delight, and he was perpetually crying aloud or bursting into song to express his joy, his joy in God the Mother Kali, who evidently existed for him as a live presence. Ramakrishna's talk was a blend of philosophical subtlety and homely parable. He spoke with a slight stammer, in the dialect of his native Bengal village, and sometimes used coarse farmyard words with the simple frankness of a peasant. By this time, his fame had spread, and many distinguished Bengalis were his constant visitors, including Keshab Chandra Sen, the leader of the Brahmo Samaj. Keshab loved and admired Ramakrishna in spite of his own reformist principles; for Ramakrishna was a ritualist and an orthodox

Hindu, and Keshab's social concern seemed to him merely an amusing and necessarily fruitless game. The world, according to a Hindu saying, is like the curly tail of a dog—how can you ever straighten it out?

So Naren went to Dakshineswar with a divided mind—half of him eager for self-dedication and devotion; the other, western-educated half, sceptical, impatient of superstition. When Naren and a few of his friends came into Ramakrishna's room, Ramakrishna asked him to sing. Naren did so. The extraordinary scene which followed can best be described in his own words:

Well, I sang that song, and then, soon after, he suddenly rose, took me by the hand and led me out on to the porch north of his room, shutting the door behind him. It was locked from the outside, so we were alone. I thought he was going to give me some advice in private. But, to my utter amazement, he began shedding tears of joy—floods of them—as he held my hand, and talking to me tenderly, as if to an old friend. "Ah!" he said, "you've come so late! How could you be so unkind—keeping me waiting so long? My ears are almost burnt off, listening to the talk of worldly people. Oh, how I've longed to unburden my heart to someone who can understand everything—my innermost experience!" He went on like this, amidst his sobbing. And then he folded his palms and addressed me solemnly, "Lord—I know you! You are Nara, the ancient sage, the incarnation of Narayana. You have come to earth to take away the sorrows of mankind...." And so forth.

I was absolutely dumbfounded by his behaviour. "Who is this man I've come to see?" I said to myself. "He must be raving mad! Why, I'm nobody—the son of Vishwanath Datta—and he dares to call me Nara!" But I kept quiet and let him go on. Presently he went back into his room and brought me out some sweets—sugar candy and butter; and he fed me with his own hands. I kept telling him, "Please give them to me—I want to share them with my friends", but it was no good. He wouldn't stop until I'd eaten all of them. Then he seized me by the hand and said, "Promise me you'll come back here alone, soon!" He was so pressing that I had to say yes. Then I went back with him to join my friends.

This was certainly a searching psychological test for an eighteen-year-old college intellectual! But Naren's intuition went much deeper than his sophistication. He was unable to dismiss Ramakrishna from his mind as a mere eccentric. If this man was mad, then even his madness was somehow holy; Naren felt that he had been in the presence of a great saint, and already he began to love him.

At their second meeting, Ramakrishna revealed himself in a quite different aspect, as a being endowed with supernatural and terrifying power. This time, Naren found him alone in his room. He greeted Naren affectionately and asked him to sit down beside him. Then, as Naren described it later:

> ... muttering something to himself, with his eyes fixed on me, he slowly drew near me... in the twinkling of an eye, he placed his right foot on my body. At his touch, I had an entirely new experience. With my eyes wide open, I saw that the walls and everything else in the room were whirling around, vanishing into nothingness; the whole universe, together with my own individuality, was about to be lost in an all-encompassing, mysterious Void! I was terribly frightened and thought I must be facing death—for the loss of my individuality meant nothing less than that to me. I couldn't control myself: I cried out, "What are you doing to me! I have my parents at home!" At this, he laughed aloud. Stroking my chest, he said, "All right, that's enough for now. Everything will come in time." The wonderful thing was, as soon as he'd said that, the whole experience came to an end. I was myself again. And everything inside and outside the room was just as it had been before.

Ramakrishna had, by his touch, taken Naren to the very brink of that superconscious experience which the Hindus call Samadhi. In Samadhi, all sense of personal identity vanishes and the real Self, the indwelling Godhead, is known. The Godhead, being a unity, is experienced as a sort of Void, in contrast to the multiplicity of objects which make up our ordinary sense consciousness. Within that Void, personal identity is lost—and loss of identity must necessarily seem, to those who are not prepared for it, like death.

For Ramakrishna, in his almost unimaginably high state of spiritual consciousness, Samadhi was a daily experience, and the awareness of God's presence never left him. Vivekananda recalls that, "I crept near him and asked him the question I had been asking others all my life: 'Do you believe in God, sir?' 'Yes,' he replied. 'Can you prove it, sir?' 'Yes.' 'How?' 'Because I see Him just as I see you here, only much more intensely.' That impressed me at once. For the first time, I found a man who dared to say that he saw God, that religion was a reality—to be felt, to be sensed in an infinitely more intense way than we can sense the world."

After this, Naren became a frequent visitor to Dakshineswar. He found himself gradually drawn into the circle of youthful disciples—most of them about his own age—whom Ramakrishna was training to follow the monastic life. But Naren did not yield to this influence easily. He kept asking himself if Ramakrishna's power could not be explained away as hypnotism. He refused, at first, to have anything to do with the worship of Kali, saying that this was mere superstition. And Ramakrishna seemed pleased at his scruples. He used to say: "Test me as the money-changers test their coins. You mustn't believe me till you've tested me thoroughly." And, in his turn, he tested Naren, ignoring him for weeks on end to find if this would stop him from coming to Dakshineswar. When it did not, Ramakrishna was delighted and congratulated him on his inner strength. "Anyone else", he said, "would have left me long ago."

Indeed, Naren's temperamental doubt is one of his most inspiring qualities. Doubt is something we have all experienced, and it should reassure us greatly that this keen observer took nothing for granted. It may even seem to us, as we read the life of Ramakrishna and see how often he granted Naren the deepest revelations, that Naren doubted too long and too much. But we must remember that Naren's faith was no facile thing. He doubted greatly because he was capable of believing greatly. For most of us, the consequences of conversion to a belief are not very far-reaching. For Naren, to believe meant absolute self-dedication to the object of his belief. No wonder he hesitated! No wonder his inner struggles were so severe!

In 1885 Ramakrishna developed cancer of the throat. As it became increasingly evident that their Master would not be with them much longer, the young disciples drew more and more closely together. Naren was their leader, together with the boy named Rakhal who later became Swami Brahmananda. One day, when Ramakrishna lay in the last stages of his illness, Naren was meditating in a room downstairs. Suddenly, he lost outward consciousness and went into Samadhi. For a moment, he was terrified and cried out, "Where is my body?" Another of the disciples thought he must be dying and ran upstairs to tell their Master. "Let him stay that way for a while;" said Ramakrishna with a smile, "he has been teasing me to give him this experience long enough." Much later, Naren came into Ramakrishna's room, full of joy and peace. "Now Mother has shown you everything," Ramakrishna told him. "But I shall keep the key. When you have done Mother's work, you will find the treasure again." This was only one of several occasions on which Ramakrishna made it clear that he had destined Naren for a mission of teaching in the world.

On 15th August 1886, Ramakrishna uttered the name of Kali in a clear ringing voice and passed into the final Samadhi. At noon next day, the doctor pronounced him dead.

The boys felt that they must hold together, and a devotee found them a house at Baranagore, about halfway between Calcutta and Dakshineswar, which they could use for their monastery. It was a dilapidated old place, with cobras under the floor, which could be rented cheaply because it was supposed to be haunted. Here they installed the ashes of Ramakrishna within a shrine, which they worshipped daily. Encouraged by Naren, they resolved to renounce the world; later they took the monastic vow in the prescribed fashion.

There were only fifteen of them. They had almost no money and few friends. Sometimes they were altogether without food, at others they lived only on boiled rice, salt, and bitter herbs. Each had two pieces of loincloth, nothing more. They owned a set of clothes in common, however, to be worn by anyone who had to go out into the city. They slept on straw mats on the floor. Yet they joked and laughed continually, sang hymns and engaged in eager philosophic discussions; they were silent only when they meditated. At all times they felt Ramakrishna's presence in their midst. Far from regarding him with awe and sadness, they could even make fun of him. A visitor to the house describes how Naren mimicked Ramakrishna going into ecstasy, while the others roared with laughter.

But gradually the boys became restless for the life of the wandering monk. With staff and begging bowl, they wandered all over India, visiting shrines and places of pilgrimage, preaching, begging, passing months of meditation in lonely huts. Sometimes they were entertained by Rajas or wealthy devotees; much more often, they shared the food of the very poor.

Such experiences were particularly valuable to Naren. During the years 1890-93 he acquired the first-hand knowledge of India's hunger, misery, nobility, and spiritual wisdom which he was to carry with him on his journey to the West. After travelling the whole length of the country he reached Cape Comorin, and here he had a vision. He saw that India had a mission in the modern world as a force for spiritual regeneration, but he also saw that this force could not become effective until India's social conditions had been radically improved. Funds must be raised for schools and hospitals; thousands of teachers and workers must be recruited and organised. It was then that he formed his decision to go to the United States in search of help. And this decision was later confirmed when the Raja of Ramnad suggested he should attend the then newly announced Chicago Parliament of Religions. Thus the specific opportunity was related to Naren's general intention. At the end of May 1893 he sailed from Bombay, via Hong Kong and Japan, to Vancouver; from there he went on by train to Chicago.

After the closing of the Parliament of Religions, Vivekananda spent nearly two whole years lecturing in various parts of the eastern and central United States, appearing chiefly in Chicago, Detroit, Boston, and New. York. By the spring of 1895 he was desperately weary and in poor health; but, characteristically, he made light of it. "Are you never serious, Swamiji?" someone once asked him, perhaps with a hint of reproach. "Oh yes", he replied, "when I have the belly-ache." He could even see the funny side of the many cranks and healers who unmercifully pestered him, hoping to steal a reflection of his glory. In his letters he refers jokingly to "the sect of Mrs. Whirlpool" and to a certain "mental healer of metaphysico-chemico-physico-religioso what not".

At the same time he met and made an impression on people of a more serious kind—Robert Ingersoll the agnostic, Nikola Tesla the inventor, Madame Calvé the singer. And, most important of all, he attracted a few students whose interest and enthusiasm were not temporary; who were prepared to dedicate the rest of their lives to the practice of his teaching. In June 1895 he was invited to bring a dozen of these to a house in Thousand Island Park on the St. Lawrence River. Here, for nearly two months, he taught them informally, as Ramakrishna had taught him and his brother-disciples. Nobody who was present ever forgot this period, and it must certainly have been much the happiest part of Vivekananda's first visit to America.

In August he sailed for France and England, returning to New York in December. It was then that, at the urgent request of his devotees, he founded the first of the Vedanta Societies in America: the Vedanta Society of New York. (Vedanta means the non-dualistic philosophy which is expounded in the Vedas, the most ancient of Hindu scriptures; and it is, of course, in line with Vivekananda s general beliefs— referred to above—that he did not call his foundation "The Ramakrishna Society".) It was then, also, that he received two academic offers, the chair of Eastern Philosophy at Harvard and a similar position at Columbia. He declined both, saying that, as a wandering monk, he could not settle down to work of this kind. In any case, he was longing to return to India. In April he sailed for England, which was to be the first stage of his journey home.

From England he took with him two of his

most faithful and energetic disciples, Captain and Mrs. Sevier—also J. J. Goodwin, an Englishman whom he had first met in America and who had become the recorder of his lectures and teachings. Later, he was followed to India by Margaret Noble, the Irishwoman who became Sister Nivedita and devoted the rest of her life to the education of Indian women and the cause of India's independence. All of these except Mrs. Sevier eventually died in India.

Vivekananda landed in Ceylon in the middle of January 1897. From there on, his journey to Calcutta was a triumphal progress. His countrymen had followed the accounts of his American lectures in the newspapers. Perhaps Vivekananda's success had sometimes been exaggerated. But they quite rightly regarded his visit to the West as a symbolic victory far exceeding in its proportions the mere amount of money he had collected for his cause or the number of disciples he had made. Indeed, one may claim that no Indian before Vivekananda had ever made Americans and Englishmen accept him on such terms—not as a subservient ally, not as an avowed opponent, but as a sincere well-wisher and friend, equally ready to teach and to learn, to ask for and to offer help. Who else had stood, as he stood, impartially between East and West, prizing the virtues and condemning the defects of both cultures? Who else could represent in his own person Young India of the nineties in synthesis with Ancient India of the Vedas? Who else could stand forth as India's champion against poverty and oppression and yet sincerely praise American idealism and British singleness of purpose? Such was Vivekananda's greatness.

In the midst of all this adulation, Vivekananda never forgot who he was: the disciple of Ramakrishna and the equal brother of his fellow monks. On 1st May 1897, he called a meeting of the monastic and householder disciples of Ramakrishna in order to establish their work on an organised basis. What Vivekananda proposed was an integration of educational, philanthropic, and religious activities; and it was thus that the Ramakrishna Mission and the Ramakrishna Math, or monastery, came into existence. The Mission went to work immediately, taking part in famine and plague relief and founding its first hospitals and schools. Brahmananda was elected as its president, and to him Vivekananda handed over all the money he had collected in America and Europe. Having done this, he was obliged to ask for a few pennies in order to take the ferryboat across the Ganga. Henceforward, he insisted on sharing the poverty of his brother monks.

The Math was consecrated some time later, at

Belur, a short distance downriver from Dakshineswar Temple, on the opposite bank of the Ganga. This Belur Math is still the chief monastery of the Ramakrishna Order, which now has nearly a hundred centres in different parts of India and neighbouring Asian lands, devoted either to the contemplative life or to social service, or to a combination of both. The Ramakrishna Mission has its own hospitals and dispensaries, its own colleges and high schools, industrial and agricultural schools, libraries and publishing houses, with monks of the Order in charge of them.

In June 1899, Vivekananda sailed for a second visit to the Western world, taking with him Nivedita and Swami Turiyananda, one of his brother monks. This time, he went by way of Europe and England, but he spent most of the next year in America. He went to California, and left Turiyananda to teach in San Francisco. It was Vivekananda's wish to found a number of Vedanta centres in the West. At the present day, there are ten centres in the United States, one in the Argentine, one in England and one in France.

By the time he returned to India, Vivekananda was a very sick man; he had said himself that he did not expect to live much longer. Yet he was happy and calm—glad, it seemed, to feel a release from the anxious energy which had driven him throughout his earlier years. Now he longed only for the peace of contemplation. Just before leaving America, he wrote a beautiful and remarkably self-revealing letter to a friend:

> I am glad I was born, glad I suffered so, glad I did make big blunders, glad to enter peace. Whether this body will fall and release me or I enter into freedom in the body, the old man is gone, gone for ever, never to come back again! Behind my work was ambition, behind my love was personality, behind my purity was fear. Now they are vanishing and I drift.

Some say that Vivekananda's departure from this life, on 4th July 1902, at the Belur Math, had the appearance of a premeditated act. For several months previously, he had been releasing himself from his various responsibilities, and training successors. His health was better. He ate his midday meal with relish, talked philosophy and went for a two-mile walk. In the evening, he passed into deep meditation, and the heart stopped beating. For hours they tried to rouse him. But his work, it seemed, was done and Ramakrishna had given him back the key to the treasure.

The best introduction to Vivekananda is not,

Title: Teachings of Swami Vivekananda
Condition: Acceptable
Description: There is handwriting, stickers or numbers inside the front cover. Corners are bent. Cover/Case has some rubbing and edgewear. Access codes, CD's, slipcovers and other accessories may not be included.
Employee: danielles

2Y6RVP003QCB

472

BP   Aisle 9   Bay 27   Shelf 5
Date Added 10/23/2024 9:10:39 AM

however, to read about him but to read him. The Swami's personality, with all its charm and force, its courageousness, its spiritual authority, its fury and its fun, comes through to you very strongly in his writings and recorded words.

In reading him, it is always well to remember that "a foolish consistency is the hobgoblin of little minds". When Emerson wrote these words in his essay on Self-Reliance, he was contrasting the "little minds" with the great minds of Jesus, Socrates, and others. No doubt Emerson would have added Vivekananda to his list if they could have met and come to know each other. But he died in 1882.

Vivekananda was the last person in the world to worry about formal consistency. He almost always spoke extempore, fired by the circumstances of the moment, addressing himself to the condition of a particular group of hearers, reacting to the intent of a certain question. That was his nature—and he was supremely indifferent if his words of today seemed to contradict those of yesterday. As a man of enlightenment, he knew that the truth is never contained in arrangements of sentences. It is within the speaker himself. If what he is is true, then words are unimportant. In this sense, Vivekananda is incapable of self-contradiction.

Vivekananda was not only a great teacher

with an international message; he was also a very great Indian, a patriot and an inspirer of his countrymen down to the present generation. But it is a mistake to think of him as a political figure, even in the best meaning of the word. First and last, he was the boy who dedicated his life to Ramakrishna. His mission was spiritual, not political or even social, in the last analysis.

The policy of the Ramakrishna Order has always been faithful to Vivekananda's intention. In the early twenties, when India's struggle with England had become intense and bitter, the Order was harshly criticised for refusing to allow its members to take part in Gandhi's Non-Cooperation Movement. But Gandhi himself never joined in this criticism. He understood perfectly that a religious body which supports a political cause—no matter how noble and just—can only compromise itself spiritually and thereby lose that very authority which is its justification for existence within human society. In 1921 Gandhi came to the Belur Math on the anniversary of Vivekananda's birthday and paid a moving tribute to him. The Swami's writings, Gandhi said, had taught him to love India even more. He reverently visited the room overlooking the Ganga in which Vivekananda spent the last months of his life.

You can visit that room today; it is still kept exactly as Vivekananda left it. But it does not seem museum-like or even unoccupied. Right next to it is the room which is used by the President of the Ramakrishna Order. There they are, dwelling side by side, the visible human authority and the invisible inspiring presence. In the life of the Belur Math, Vivekananda still lives and is as much a participant in its daily activities as any of its monks.

June 1960   CHRISTOPHER ISHERWOOD

TEACHINGS OF
SWAMI VIVEKANANDA

I

ATMAN OR THE SELF

1. The Background, the Reality, of everyone is that same Eternal, Ever Blessed, Ever Pure, and Ever Perfect One. It is the Atman, the Soul, in the saint and the sinner, in the happy and the miserable, in the beautiful and the ugly, in men and in animals; it is the same throughout. It is the Shining One. (II. 168).

2. Here I stand and if I shut my eyes, and try to conceive my existence, "I", "I", "I",— what is the idea before me? The idea of a body. Am I, then, nothing but a combination of material substances? The Vedas declare, "No". I am a spirit living in a body. I am not the body. The body will die, but I shall not die. Here am I in this body; it will fall, but I shall go on living. (I. 7-8.)

3. The Vedas say the whole world is a mixture of independence and dependence, of freedom and slavery, but through it all shines the soul independent, immortal, pure, perfect, holy. For if it is independent, it cannot perish, as death is but a change, and depends upon conditions; if independent, it must be perfect, for imperfection is again but a condition, and therefore dependent. And this immortal and perfect

soul must be the same in the highest God as well as in the humblest man, the difference between them being only in the degree in which this soul manifests itself. (I. 330.)

4. It cannot be that the soul knows, but it *is* knowledge. It cannot be that the soul is happy, it *is* happiness itself. That which is happy, has borrowed its happiness; that which has knowledge, has received its knowledge; and that which has relative existence, has only a reflected existence. (II. 216.)

5. That very thing which we now see as the universe, will appear to us as God (Absolute), and that very God who has so long been external will appear to be internal, as our own Self. (I. 404.)

6. There is no change whatsoever in the Soul—Infinite, Absolute, Eternal, Knowledge, Bliss, and Existence. (I. 421.)

7. If there is one common doctrine that runs through all our apparently fighting and contradictory sects, it is that all glory, power and purity are within the soul already; only according to Ramanuja the soul contracts and expands at times, and according to Shankara, it comes under a delusion. Never mind these differences. All admit the truth that the power is there—potential or manifest, it is there—and the sooner you believe that, the better for you. (III. 284.)

ATMAN OR THE SELF

8. The feeling of independence which possesses us all, shows there is something in us besides mind and body. The soul that reigns within is independent, and creates the desire for freedom. (IV. 190.)

9. Each soul is a star, and all stars are set in that infinite azure, that eternal sky, the Lord. There is the root, the reality, the real individuality of each and all. Religion began with the search after some of these stars that had passed beyond our horizon, and ended in finding them all in God, and ourselves in the same place. (V. 69).

10. Know then, that thou art He, and model your whole life accordingly, and he who knows this and models his life accordingly, will no more grovel in darkness. (II. 237.)

11. This truth about the soul is first to be heard. If you have heard, it, think about it. Once you have done that, meditate upon it. No more vain arguments! Satisfy yourself once that you are the infinite spirit. If that is true, it must be nonsense that you are the body. You are the Self, and that must be realised. Spirit must see itself as spirit. Now the spirit is seeing itself as the body. That must stop. The moment you begin to realise that, you are released. (IV. 245.)

12. As we cannot know except through effects that we have eyes, so we cannot see the Self

except by Its effects. It cannot be brought down to the low plane of sense-perception. It is the condition of everything in the universe, though Itself unconditioned. (VI. 84).

13. It is not for the sake of the husband that the wife loves the husband, but for the sake of the Atman that she loves the husband, because she loves the Self. None loves the wife for the sake of the wife, but it is because he loves the Self that he loves the wife. None loves the children for the children; but because one loves the Self, therefore one loves the children. None loves wealth on account of the wealth; but because one loves the Self, therefore one loves wealth. None loves the Brahmana for the sake of the Brahmana; but because one loves the Self, one loves the Brahmana. So, none loves the Kshatriya for the sake of the Kshatriya, but because one loves the Self. Neither does any one love the world on account of the world, but because one loves the Self. None, similarly, loves the gods on account of the gods, but because one loves the Self. None loves a thing for that thing's sake; but it is for the Self that one loves it. This Self, therefore, is to be heard, reasoned about, and meditated upon. (II. 416-17.)

14. Within there is the lion—the eternally pure, illumined and ever free Atman; and directly one realises It through meditation and concen-

ATMAN OR THE SELF

tration, this world of Maya vanishes. It is equally present in all, and the more one practises, the quicker does the Kundalini (the "coiled-up" power) awaken in one. When this power reaches the head, one's vision is unobstructed—one realises the Atman. (VII. 253.)

15. "Whom the ignorant worship, Him I preach unto thee."

This one and only God is the "Knownest" of the known. He is the one thing we see everywhere. All know their own Self, all know, "I am", even animals. All we know is the projection of the Self. (VII. 93).

16. That Self-existent One is far removed from the organs. The organs or instruments see outwards, but the self-existing One, the Self, is seen inwards. You must remember the qualification that is required: the desire to know this Self by turning the eyes inwards. (II. 411.)

17. Those who are evil-doers, whose minds are not peaceful, can never see the Light. It is to those who are true in heart, pure in deed, whose senses are controlled, that this Self manifests itself. (II. 169.)

18. This Atman is not to be reached by too much talking, nor is it to be reached by the power of the intellect, nor by much study of the scriptures. (III. 345.)

19. After long searches here and there, in

temples and churches, in earths and in heavens, at last you come back, completing the circle from where you started, to your own soul and find that He, for whom you have been seeking all over the world, for whom you have been weeping and praying in churches and temples, on whom you were looking as the mystery of all mysteries shrouded in the clouds, is nearest of the near, is your own Self, the reality of your life, body, and soul. (II. 81-82.)

II

BHAKTI OR THE LOVE OF GOD

1. Bhakti-Yoga is a real, genuine search after the Lord, a search beginning, continuing and ending in Love. One single moment of the madness of extreme love to God brings us eternal freedom. (III. 31.)

2. "Bhakti is intense love to God." "When a man gets it he loves all, hates none; he becomes satisfied for ever." "This love cannot be reduced to any earthly benefit," because so long as worldly desires last that kind of love does not come. (III. 31.)

3. "Bhakti is greater than Karma, greater than Yoga, because these are intended for an object in view, while Bhakti is its own fruition, its own means and its own end." (III. 31-32.)

4. The one great advantage of Bhakti is that it is the easiest, and the most natural way to reach the great divine end in view; its great disadvantage is that in its lower forms it oftentimes degenerates into hideous fanaticism. The fanatical crew in Hinduism, or Mohammedanism, or Christianity, have always been almost exclusively recruited from these worshippers on the lower planes of Bhakti. (III. 32.)

5. That singleness of attachment to a loved

object, without which no genuine love can grow, is very often also the cause of the denunciation of everything else. All the weak and undeveloped minds in every religion or country have only one way of loving their own ideal, i.e. by hating every other ideal. Herein is the explanation of why the same man who is so lovingly attached to his own ideal of God, so devoted to his own ideal of religion, becomes a howling fanatic as soon as he sees or hears anything of any other ideal. (III. 32.)

6. In every mind, utility... is conditioned by its own peculiar wants. To men, therefore, who never rise higher than eating, drinking, begetting progeny, and dying, the only gain is in sense-enjoyments; and they must wait and go through many more births and reincarnations to learn to feel even the faintest necessity for anything higher. But those to whom the eternal interests of the soul are of much higher value than the fleeting interests of this mundane life, to whom the gratification of the senses is but like the thoughtless play of the baby, to them, God and the love of God form the highest and the only utility of human existence. (III. 43.)

7. There is Bhakti within you, only a veil of lust-and-wealth covers it, and as soon as that is removed Bhakti will manifest by itself. (V. 314.)

8. One way for attaining Bhakti is by repeat-

ing the name of God a number of times. Mantras have effect—the mere repetition of words.... To obtain Bhakti, seek the company of holy men who have Bhakti, and read books like the Gita and the *Imitation of Christ;* always think of the attributes of God. (VI. 122-23.)

9. But theorising about God will not do; we must love and work. Give up the world and all worldly things, especially while the "plant" is tender. Day and night think of nothing else as far as possible. The daily necessary thoughts can all be thought through God. Eat to Him, drink to Him, sleep to Him, see Him in all. Talk of God to others; this is most beneficial. (VII. 9.)

10. Get the mercy of God and of His greatest children; these are the two chief ways to God. The company of these children of Light is very hard to get; five minutes in their company will change a whole life, and if you really want it enough, one will come to you. The presence of those who love God makes a place holy, "such is the glory of the children of the Lord". They are He; and when they speak, their words are Scriptures. The place where they have been becomes filled with their vibrations, and those going there feel them and have a tendency to become holy also. (VII. 10.)

11. Bhakti-Yoga does not say "give up"; it

only says "Love; love the Highest"; and everything low naturally falls off from him, the object of whose love is this Highest. (III. 74)

12. In Bhakti-Yoga the first essential is to want God honestly and intensely. We want everything but God, because our ordinary desires are fulfilled by the external world. So long as our needs are confined within the limits of the physical universe, we do not feel any need for God; it is only when we have had hard blows in our lives and are disappointed with everything here that we feel the need for something higher; then we seek God. (VII. 83.)

13. Bhakti is not destructive; it teaches that all our faculties may become means to reach salvation. We must turn them all towards God and give to Him that love which is usually wasted on the fleeting objects of sense. (VII. 83.)

14. Bhakti differs from your Western idea of religion in that Bhakti admits no elements of fear, no Being to be appeased or propitiated. There are even Bhaktas, who worship God as their own child, so that there may remain no feeling even of awe or reverence. There can be no fear in true love, and so long as there is the least fear, Bhakti cannot even begin. In Bhakti there is also no place for begging or bargaining with God. The idea of asking God for anything is sacrilege to a Bhakta. He will not pray for

health or wealth or even to go to heaven (VII. 83.)

15. We all have to begin as dualists in the religion of love. God is to us a separate Being, and we feel ourselves to be separate beings also. Love then comes in the middle, and man begins to approach God, and God also comes nearer and nearer to man. Man takes up all the various relationships of life, as father, as mother, as son, as friend, as master, as lover, and projects them on his ideal of love, on his God. To him God exists as all these, and the last point of his progress is reached when he feels that he has become absolutely merged in the object of his worship. (III. 100.)

16. We all begin with love for ourselves and the unfair claims of the little self make even love selfish; at last, however, comes the full blaze of light, in which this little self is seen to have become one with the Infinite. Man himself is transfigured in the presence of this Light of Love, and he realises at last the beautiful and inspiring truth that Love, the Lover, and the Beloved are one. (III. 100.)

17. The path of devotion is natural and pleasant. Philosophy is taking the mountain stream back to its source by force. It is a quicker method but very hard. Philosophy says, "Check everything." Devotion says, "Give up all to the

stream, have eternal self-surrender." It is a longer way, but easier and happier. (VII. 44.)

18. Leave inimical thoughts aside if you want to have permanent Bhakti. Hatred is a thing which greatly impedes the course of Bhakti, and the man who hates none reaches God. (III. 358.)

19. If a man does not get food one day, he is troubled; if his son dies how agonising it is to him! The true Bhakta feels the same pangs in his heart when he yearns for God. The great quality of Bhakti is that it cleanses the mind, and the firmly established Bhakti for the Supreme Lord is alone sufficient to purify the mind. (III. 358.)

20. Of all renunciations, the most natural, so to say, is that of the Bhakti-Yogi. Here, there is no violence, nothing to give up, nothing to tear off, as it were, from ourselves, nothing from which we have violently to separate ourselves; the Bhakta's renunciation is easy, smooth, flowing, and as natural as the things around us. (III. 71.)

21. "In this evanescent world, where everything is falling to pieces, we have to make the highest use of what time we have," says the Bhakta; and really the highest use of life is to hold it at the service of all beings. (III. 84.)

22. It is the horrible body-idea that breeds all the selfishness in the world, just this one

BHAKTI OR THE LOVE OF GOD

delusion that we are wholly the body we own, and that we must by all possible means try our very best to preserve and please it. If you know that you are positively other than your body, you have then none to fight with or struggle against; you are dead to all ideals of selfishness. So the Bhakta declares that we have to hold ourselves as if we are altogether dead to all the things of the world; and that is indeed self-surrender. Let things come as they may. This is the meaning of "Thy will be done"; not going about fighting and struggling and thinking all the while that God wills all our own weaknesses and worldly ambitions. (III. 84)

23. "Lord, they build high temples in your name; they make gifts in your name; I am poor; I have nothing; so I take this body of mine and place it at your feet. Do not give me up, O Lord." Such is the prayer proceeding out of the depths of the Bhakta's heart. To him who has experienced it, this eternal sacrifice of the self unto the Beloved Lord is higher by far than all wealth and power, than even all soaring thoughts of renown and enjoyment. (III. 84.)

24. The peace of the Bhakta's calm resignation is a peace that passeth all understanding, and is of incomparable value. (III. 84.)

25. When the devotee has reached this point he is no more impelled to ask whether God can

be demonstrated or not, whether He is omnipotent and omniscient, or not. To him He is only the God of Love; He is the highest ideal of love, and that is sufficient for all his purposes; He, as love, is self-evident; it requires no proof to demonstrate the existence of the beloved to the lover. The magistrate-Gods of other forms of religion may require a good deal of proof to prove them, but the Bhakta does not and cannot think of such Gods at all. To him God exists entirely as love. (III. 91-92.)

26. The perfected Bhakta no more goes to see God in temples and churches; he knows no place where he will not find Him. He finds Him in the temple as well as out of the temple; he finds Him in the saint's saintliness as well as in the wicked man's wickedness, because he has Him already seated in glory in his own heart, as the one Almighty, inextinguishable Light of Love, which is ever shining and eternally present. (III. 92-93.)

27. The Bhakta at last comes to this that love itself is God and nothing else. Where should man go to prove the existence of God? Love was the most visible of all visible things. It was the force that was moving the sun, the moon and the stars, manifesting itself in men, women and in animals, everywhere and in everything. It was expressed in material forces as gravita-

tion and so on. It was everywhere, in every atom, manifesting everywhere. It was that Infinite Love, the only motive power of this universe, visible everywhere, and this was God Himself. (III. 392.)

28. "I may know that I am He, yet will I take myself away from Him and become different, so that I may enjoy the Beloved." That is what the Bhakta says. (III. 99.)

29. I know one whom the world used to call mad, and this was his answer: "My friends, the whole world is a lunatic asylum; some are mad after worldly love, some after name, some after fame, some after money, some after salvation and going to heaven. In this big lunatic asylum I am also mad, I am mad after God. You are mad; so am I. I think my madness is after all the best." The true Bhakta's love is this burning madness, before which everything else vanishes for him. The whole universe is to him full of love and love alone; that is how it seems to the lover. So when a man has this love in him, he becomes eternally blessed, eternally happy; this blessed madness of divine love alone can cure for ever the disease of the world that is in us. (III. 99-100.)

30. Men are ever running after wives, and wealth, and fame in this world; sometimes they are hit very hard on the head, and they find out

what this world really is. No one in this world can really love anything but God. Man finds out that human love is all hollow. Men cannot love though they talk of it. The wife says, she loves her husband, and kisses him; but as soon as he dies the first thing she thinks about is the bank account, and what she shall do the next day. The husband loves the wife, but when she becomes sick, and loses her beauty, or becomes haggard, or makes a mistake, he ceases to care for her. All the love of the world is hypocrisy and hollowness. (IV. 15.)

31. With love there is no painful reaction; love only brings a reaction of bliss; if it does not, it is not love; it is mistaking something else for love. When you have succeeded in loving your husband, your wife, your children, the whole world, the universe, in such a manner that there is no reaction of pain or jealousy, no selfish feeling, then you are in a fit state to be unattached. (I. 58.)

32. *Q.*—Then is it impossible for householders to realise God through that path of love, worshipping God as one's own husband or lover and considering oneself as His spouse?

A.—With a few exceptions; for ordinary householders it is impossible no doubt. And why lay so much stress on this delicate path, above all others? Are there no other relationships by which to worship God, except this Madhura idea of love? Why not follow the four other paths, and take the name of the Lord with all your heart? Let the heart be opened first, and all else will follow of itself. But know this for certain, that Prema cannot come while there is lust. Why not try first to get rid of carnal desires? You will say—"How is that possible? —I am a householder." Nonsense! Because one is a householder, does it mean that one should be a personification of incontinence, or that one has to live in marital relations all one's life? And, after all, how unbecoming of a man to make of himself a woman, so that he may practise this Madhura love! (V. 346.)

33. We accept God not because we really want Him, but because we have need of him for selfish purposes. Love is something absolutely unselfish, that which has no thought beyond the glorification and adoration of the object upon which our affections are bestowed. It is a quality which bows down and worships and asks nothing in return. Merely to love is the sole request that true love has to ask. (VIII. 201.)

34. Then alone a man loves when he finds that the object of his love is not any low, little mortal thing. Then alone a man loves when he finds that the object of his love is not a clod of earth, but is the veritable God Himself. The

wife will love the husband the more when she thinks that the husband is God Himself. The husband will love the wife the more when he knows that the wife is God Himself. The mother will love the children more, who thinks that the children are God Himself. That man will love his greatest enemy, who knows that that very enemy is God Himself. That man will love a holy man, who knows that the holy man is God Himself, and that very man will also love the unholiest of men because he knows the background of that unholiest of men is even He, the Lord. (II. 286.)

35. The absence of the thought of self is the essential characteristic of the love for God. Religion nowadays has become a mere hobby and fashion. People go to church like a flock of sheep. They do not embrace God because they need Him. Most persons are unconscious atheists who self-complacently think that they are devout believers. (VIII. 203.)

III

BRAHMAN OR THE SUPREME REALITY

1. Brahman is the last generalisation to which we can come. It has no attributes but is Existence, Knowledge, and Bliss—Absolute. Existence, we have seen, is the very ultimate generalisation which the human mind can come to. Knowledge does not mean the knowledge we have, but the essence of that, which is expressing itself in the course of evolution in human beings or in other animals, as knowledge. The essence of that knowledge is meant, the ultimate fact beyond, if I may be allowed to say so, even consciousness. That is what is meant by Knowledge and what we see in the universe as the essential unity of things. (I. 372-73.)

2. The Brahman, the God of the Vedanta, has nothing outside of Himself; nothing at all. All indeed is He; He is in the universe; He is the universe Himself. "Thou art the man, Thou art the woman, Thou art the young man walking in the pride of youth, Thou art the old man tottering in his step." (I. 374.)

3. Brahman is Sat-Chit-Ananda—the Absolute Existence-Knowledge-Bliss. The phrase Sat-Chit-Ananda means—Sat, i.e. Existence, Chit, i.e.

Consciousness, or Knowledge, and Ananda, i.e. Bliss, which is the same as Love. There is no controversy between the Bhakta and the Jnani regarding the Sat aspect of Brahman. Only the Jnanis lay greater stress on His aspect of Chit, or Knowledge, while the Bhaktas keep the aspect of Ananda, or Love, more in view. But no sooner is the essence of Chit realised than the essence of Ananda is also realised. Because what is Chit is verily the same as Ananda. (V. 385.)

4. We sometimes indicate a thing by describing its surroundings. When we say "Sat-Chit-Ananda" (Existence-Knowledge-Bliss) we are merely indicating the shores of an indescribable Beyond. Nor can we say "is" about it, for that too is relative. Any imagination, any concept is in vain. Neti, neti ("not this, not this") is all that can be said, for even to think is to limit and so to lose. (VII. 74.)

5. Brahman is one, but is at the same time appearing to us as many, on the relative plane. Name and form are at the root of this relativity. For instance, what do you find when you abstract name and form from a jar? Only earth, which is its essence. Similarly, through delusion you are thinking of and seeing a jar, a cloth, a monastery and so on. The phenomenal world depends on this nescience which obstructs knowledge and which has no real existence. One sees

variety such as wife, children, body, mind—only in the world created by nescience by means of name and form. As soon as this nescience is removed, the realisation of Brahman which eternally exists is the result. (VII. 163.)

6. You are also that undivided Brahman. This very moment you can realise it, if you think yourself truly and absolutely to be so. It is all mere want of direct perception.... Being again and again entangled in the intricate maze of delusion and hard hit by sorrows and afflictions, the eye will turn of itself to one's own real nature, the Inner Self. It is owing to the presence of this desire for bliss in the heart, that man, getting hard shocks, one after another, turns his eye inwards—to his own Self. A time is sure to come to everyone, without exception, when he will do so—to one it may be in this life, to another after thousands of incarnations. (V. 393.)

7. All this universe was in Brahman, and it was, as it were, projected out of Him, and has been moving on, to go back to the source from which it was projected, like the electricity which comes out of the dynamo, completes the circuit, and returns to it. The same is the case with the soul. Projected from Brahman, it passed through all sorts of vegetable and animal forms, and at last it is in man, and man is the nearest approach to Brahman. To go back to Brahman from which

we have been projected is the great struggle of life. (II. 258-59.)

8. He who is beyond the senses, beyond all touch, beyond all form, beyond all taste, the Unchangeable, the Infinite, beyond even intelligence, the Indestructible—knowing Him alone, we are safe from the jaws of death. (II. 410.)

IV

BUDDHA

1. Shakya Muni came not to destroy, but he was the fulfilment, the logical conclusion, the logical development of the religion of the Hindus. (I. 21.)

2. I would like to see moral men like Gautama Buddha, who did not believe in a Personal God or a personal soul, never asked about them, but was a perfect agnostic, and yet was ready to lay down his life for anyone, and worked all his life for the good of all, and thought only for the good of all. Well has it been said by his biographer, in describing his birth, that he was born for the good of the many, as a blessing to the many. He did not go to the forest to meditate for his own salvation; he felt that the world was burning, and that he must find a way out. "Why is there so much misery in the world?"—was the one question that dominated his whole life. (II. 352.)

3. Buddha was a great Vedantist (for Buddhism was really only an offshoot of Vedanta), and Shankara is often called a "hidden Buddhist".... Buddha never bowed down to anything, neither Veda, nor caste, nor priest, nor custom. He fearlessly reasoned so far as reason

could take him. Such a fearless search for truth and such love for every living thing the world has never seen. (VII. 59.)

4. What was in this country before Buddha's advent? Only a number of religious principles recorded on bundles of palm leaves—and those too known only to a few. It was Lord Buddha who brought them down to the practical field, and showed how to apply them in the everyday life of the people. In a sense, he was the living embodiment of true Vedanta. (VII. 118-19.)

5. To help the suffering world was the gigantic task to which Buddha gave prominence, brushing aside for the time being almost all other phases of religion; yet he had to spend years in self-searching, to realise the great truth of the utter hollowness of clinging to a selfish individuality. A more unselfish and untiring worker is beyond our sanguine imagination, yet, who had harder struggles to realise the meaning of things, than he? It holds good in all times that the greater the work, the more must have been the power of realisation behind. (IV. 283.)

6. Listen to Buddha's message—a tremendous message. It has a place in our heart. Says Buddha: "Root out selfishness, and everything that makes you selfish. Have neither wife, child, nor family. Be not of the world; become perfectly unselfish." A worldly man thinks he will be

unselfish, but when he looks at the face of his wife it makes him selfish. The mother thinks she will be perfectly unselfish, but she looks at her baby, and immediately selfishness comes. So with everything in this world. As soon as selfish desires arise, as soon as some selfish pursuit is followed, immediately the whole man, the real man, is gone: he is like a brute, he is a slave, he forgets his fellow men. No more does he say, "You first and I afterwards", but it is "I first and let every one else look out for himself". (IV. 131-32.)

7. Buddha is the only prophet who said, "I do not care to know your various theories about God. What is the use of discussing all subtle doctrines about the soul? Do good and be good And this will take you to freedom and to whatever truth there is". (I. 117.)

8. Buddha was the first who dared to say, "Believe not because some old manuscripts are produced, believe not because it is your national belief, because you have been made to believe it from your childhood; but reason it all out, and after you have analysed it, then, if you find that it will do good to one and all, believe it, live up to it, and help others to live up to it". (I. 117.)

9. There were other great men, who all said they were the Incarnations of God Himself, and that those who would believe in them would go to heaven. But what did Buddha say with his

dying breath? "None can help you; help yourself; work out your own salvation". (IV. 136.)

10. He said about himself, "Buddha is the name of infinite knowledge, infinite as the sky; I, Gautama, have reached that state; you will reach that too if you struggle for it". (IV. 136.)

11. Bereft of all motive power, Buddha did not want to go to heaven, did not want money; he gave up his throne and everything else, and went about begging his bread through the streets of India, preaching for the good of men and animals with a heart as wide as the ocean. He was the only man who was ever ready to give up his life for animals, to stop a sacrifice. He once said to a king, "If the sacrifice of a lamb helps you to go to heaven, sacrificing a man will help you better, so sacrifice me." The king was astonished. (IV. 136.)

12. To many the path becomes easier, if they believe in God. But the life of Buddha shows that even a man who does not believe in God, has no metaphysics, belongs to no sect, and does not go to any church, or temple, and is a confessed materialist, even he can attain to the highest. We have no right to judge him. I wish I had one infinitesimal part of Buddha's heart. Buddha may or may not have believed in God; that does not matter to me. He reached the

same state of perfection to which others come by Bhakti—love of God, Yoga, or Jnana. (IV. 136.)

13. He alone can be religious who dares say, as the mighty Buddha once said under the Bo-tree.... When the temptation came to him to give up his search after truth, to go back to the world and live the old life of fraud, calling things by wrong names, telling lies to oneself and to everybody, he, the giant, conquered it and said, "Death is better than a vegetating ignorant life; it is better to die on the battlefield than to live a life of defeat". (II. 124.)

14. It was the Great Buddha, who never cared for the dualist gods, and who has been called an atheist and materialist, who yet was ready to give up his body for a poor goat. That Man set in motion the highest moral ideas any nation can have. Wherever there is a moral code, it is a ray of light from that Man. (II. 143.)

15. Buddha was one of the Sannyasins of the Vedanta. He started a new sect, just as others are started even today. The ideas which now are called Buddhism were not his. They were much more ancient. He was a great man who gave the ideas power. The unique element in Buddhism was its social element. (V. 309.)

16. Buddha was more brave and sincere than any teacher. He said: "Believe no book; the Vedas are all humbug. If they agree with me,

so much the better for the books. I am the greatest book; sacrifice and prayer are useless." Buddha was the first human being to give to the world a complete system of morality. He was good for good's sake, he loved for love's sake. (VII. 40-41.)

17. What Buddha did was to break wide open the gates of that very religion which was confined in the Upanishads to a particular caste. What special greatness does his theory of Nirvana confer on him? His greatness lies in his unrivalled sympathy. The high orders of Samadhi etc. that lend gravity to his religion, are almost all there in the Vedas; what are absent there are his intellect and heart, which have never since been paralleled throughout the history of the world. (VI. 225-26.)

V

BUDDHISM

1. On the philosophic side the disciples of the Great Master dashed themselves against the eternal rocks of the Vedas and could not crush them, and on the other side they took away from the nation that eternal God to which every one, man or woman, clings so fondly. And the result was that Buddhism had to die a natural death in India. (I. 22.)

2. Buddha brought the Vedanta to light, gave it to the people, and saved India. A thousand years after his death a similar state of things again prevailed. The mob, the masses, various races, had been converted to Buddhism; naturally the teachings of Buddha became in time degenerated, because most of the people were ignorant. Buddhism taught no God, no Ruler of the universe, so gradually the masses brought their gods, devils, and hobgoblins, out again, and a tremendous hotchpotch was made of Buddhism in India. (II. 139.)

3. The earlier Buddhists in their rage against the killing of animals, had denounced the sacrifices of the Vedas; and these sacrifices used to be held in every house. There was a fire burning, and that was all the paraphernalia of worship.

These sacrifices were obliterated, and in their place came gorgeous temples, gorgeous ceremonies, and gorgeous priests and all that you see in modern times. I smile when I read books written by some modern people who ought to have known better, that Buddha was the destroyer of Brahminical idolatry. Little do they know that Buddhism created Brahminism and idolatry in India. (III. 263-64.)

4. I have every respect and veneration for Lord Buddha, but mark my words, the spread of Buddhism was less owing to the doctrines and the personality of the great preacher, than to the temples that were built, the idols that were erected, and the gorgeous ceremonies that were put before the nation. Thus Buddhism progressed. The little fireplaces in the houses, in which the people poured their libations were not strong enough to hold their own against the gorgeous temples and ceremonies, but later on the whole thing degenerated. (III. 217.)

5. The result of Buddha's constant inveighing against a personal God was the introduction of idols into India. In the Vedas they knew them not, because they saw God everywhere, but the reaction against the loss of God as Creator and Friend was to make idols, and Buddha became an idol—so too with Jesus. The range of idols

is from wood and stone to Jesus and Buddha, but we must have idols. (VII. 21-22.)

6. The Vedanta has no quarrel with Buddhism. The idea of the Vedanta is to harmonise all. With the Northern Buddhists we have no quarrel at all. But the Burmese and Siamese and all the Southern Buddhists say that there is a phenomenal world, and ask what right we have to create a noumenal world behind this. The answer of the Vedanta is that this is a false statement. The Vedanta never contended that there is a noumenal and a phenomenal world. There is one. Seen through the senses it is phenomenal, but it is really the noumenal all the time. The man who sees the rope does not see the snake. It is either the rope or the snake, but never the two. So the Buddhistic statement of our position, that we believe there are two worlds, is entirely false. They have the right to say it is the phenomenal if they like, but no right to contend that other men have not the right to say it is the noumenal. (V. 279-80.)

7. The Buddhist tenet, "Non-killing is supreme virtue", is very good, but in trying to enforce it upon all by legislation without paying any heed to the capacities of the people at large, Buddhism has brought ruin upon India. I have come across many a "religious hypocrite" in India, who fed ants with sugar, and at the same time would not

hesitate to bring ruin on his own brother for the sake of "filthy lucre"! (V. 401.)

8. The master says that selfishness is the great curse of the world; that we are selfish and that therein is the curse. There should be no motive for selfishness. You are (like a river) passing (on) —a continuous phenomenon. Have no God; have no soul; stand on your feet and do good for good's sake—neither for fear of punishment nor for (the sake of) going anywhere. Stand sane and motiveless. (III. 529.)

9. The great majority of the adherents of Northern Buddhism believe in Mukti and are really Vedantists. Only the Ceylonese accept Nirvana as annihilation. (VII. 94.)

VI

CHRIST

1. That soul is strong that has become one with the Lord; none else is strong. In your own Bible, what do you think was the cause of that strength of Jesus of Nazareth, that immense, infinite strength which laughed at traitors, and blessed those that were willing to murder him? It was that, "I and my Father are one"; it was that prayer, "Father, just as I am one with you, so make them one with me". (I. 381.)

2. It is the Man who said, "I and my Father are one", whose power has descended unto millions. For thousands of years it has worked for good. And we know that the same Man, because he was a non-dualist, was merciful to others. To the masses who could not conceive of anything higher than a Personal God, he said, "Pray to your Father in heaven." To others who could grasp a higher idea, he said: "I am the vine, ye are the branches," but to his disciples to whom he revealed himself more fully, he proclaimed the highest truth, "I and my Father are one". (II. 142-43.)

3. We have read different stories that have been written about him; we know the scholars and their writings, and the higher criticism; and

we know all that has been done by study. We are not here to discuss how much of the New Testament is true, we are not here to discuss how much of that life is historical. It does not matter at all whether the New Testament was written within five hundred years of his birth; nor does it matter, even, how much of that life is true. But there is something behind it, something we want to imitate. To tell a lie, you have to imitate a truth, and that truth is a fact. You cannot imitate that which you never perceived. But there must have been a nucleus, a tremendous power that came down; a marvellous manifestation of spiritual power; and of that we are speaking. It stands there. Therefore, we are not afraid of all the criticisms of the scholars. If I, as an Oriental have to worship Jesus of Nazareth, there is only one way left to me, that is, to worship him as God and nothing else. (IV. 146-47.)

4. The great secret of true success, of true happiness, then, is this: the man who asks for no return, the perfectly unselfish man, is the most successful. It seems to be a paradox: do we not know that every man who is unselfish in life gets cheated, gets hurt? Apparently, yes. "Christ was unselfish, and yet he was crucified." True; but we know that his unselfishness is the reason, the cause of a great victory—the crown-

CHRIST

ing of millions upon millions of lives with the blessings of true success. (II. 4-5.)

5. Nowadays it is very hard even to talk of renunciation. It was said of me in America that I was a man who came out of a land that had been dead and buried for five thousand years, and talked of renunciation. So says perhaps the English philosopher. Yet it is true that that is the only path to religion. Renounce and give up. What did Christ say? "He that loseth his life for my sake shall find it." Again and again did he preach renunciation as the only way to perfection. (II. 100.)

6. "Blessed are the pure in heart for they shall see God." "The Kingdom of Heaven is within you." Where goest thou to seek for the kingdom of God? asks Jesus of Nazareth, when it is there, within you. Cleanse the spirit, and it is there. It is already yours. How can you get what is not yours? It is yours by right. You are the heirs of immortality, sons of the Eternal Father. (IV. 149.)

7. Let the Churches preach doctrines, theories, philosophies to their heart's content, but when it comes to worship, the real practical part of religion, it should be as Jesus says, "When thou prayest, enter into thy closet, and when thou hast shut thy door, pray to thy Father which is in secret". (IV. 56-57.)

8. The three years of his ministry were like

one compressed, concentrated age, which it has taken nineteen hundred years to unfold, and who knows how much longer it will yet take! Little men like you and me are simply the recipients of just a little energy. A few minutes, a few hours, a few years at best, are enough to spend it all, to stretch it out, as it were, to its fullest strength, and then we are gone for ever. But mark this giant that came: centuries and ages pass, yet the energy that he left upon the world is not yet stretched, nor yet expended to its full. It goes on adding new vigour as the ages roll on. (IV. 138-39.)

9. The Trinitarian Christ is elevated above us; the Unitarian Christ is merely a mortal man; neither can help us. The Christ who is the Incarnation of God, who has not forgotten His divinity, that Christ can help us, in Him there is no imperfection. These Incarnations are always conscious of their own divinity; they know it from their birth. They are like the actors whose play is over, but who, after their work is done, return to please others. These great ones are untouched by aught of earth; they assume our form and limitations for a time in order to teach us, but in reality they are never limited, they are ever free. (VII. 4.)

10. How can you make the spirit pure? By renunciation. A rich young man asked Jesus,

CHRIST

"Good Master, what shall I do that I may inherit eternal life?" And Jesus said unto him, "One thing thou lackest; go thy way, sell whatsoever thou hast, and give to the poor, and thou shalt have treasures in heaven: and come, take up thy cross, and follow me". (IV. 149.)

VII

CHRISTIANITY

1. The most profound and noble ideals of Christianity were never understood in Europe because the ideas and images used by the writers of the Bible were foreign to it.... Through all the myths and mythologies by which it is surrounded it is no wonder that the people get very little of the beautiful religion of Jesus, and no wonder that they have made of it a modern shopkeeping religion. (I. 321-22.)

2. "Watch and pray, for the Kingdom of Heaven is at hand," which means, purify your mind and be ready! And that spirit never dies. You recollect that the Christians are, even in the darkest days, even in the most superstitious Christian countries, always trying to prepare themselves, for the coming of the Lord, by trying to help others, building hospitals, and so on. So long as the Christians keep to that ideal, their religion lives. (II. 372.)

3. One of the chief distinctions between the Hindu and the Christian religion is that the Christian religion teaches that each human soul had its beginning, at its birth into this world; whereas the Hindu religion asserts that the Spirit of man is an emanation of the Eternal

Being, and had no more a beginning than God Himself. Innumerable have been and will be its manifestations in its passage from one personality to another, subject to the great law of spiritual evolution, until it reaches perfection, when there is no more change. (IV. 188-89.)

4. So we find that in almost every religion these are the three primary things which we have in the worship of God—forms or symbols, names, God-men. All religions have these, but you find that they want to fight with each other. One says, "My name is the only name; my form is the only form; and my God-men are the only God-men in the world; yours are simply myths." In modern times, Christian clergymen have become a little kinder, and they allow that in the older religions, the different forms of worship were foreshadowings of Christianity, which of course, they consider, is the only true form. God tested Himself in older times, tested His powers by getting these things into shape which culminated in Christianity. This, at least, is a great advance. Fifty years ago they would not have said even that; nothing was true except their own religion. This idea is not limited to any religion, nation, or class of persons; people are always thinking that the only right thing to be done by others is what they themselves are doing. And it is here that the study of different religions helps us. It

shows us that the same thoughts that we have been calling ours, and ours alone, were present hundreds of years ago, in others, and sometimes even in better form of expression than our own. (II. 42-43.)

5. All religions are, at bottom, alike. This is so, although the Christian Church, like the Pharisee in the parable, thanks God that it alone is right and thinks that all other religions are wrong and in need of Christian light. Christianity must become tolerant before the world will be willing to unite with the Christian Church in a common charity. God has not left Himself without a witness in any heart, and men, especially men who follow Jesus Christ, should be willing to admit this. In fact, Jesus Christ was willing to admit every good man to the family of God. It is not the man who believes a certain something, but the man who does the will of the Father in heaven, who is right. On this basis—being right and doing right—the whole world can unite. (V. 292-93.)

VIII

CONCENTRATION

1. How has all the knowledge in the world been gained but by the concentration of the powers of the mind? The world is ready to give up its secrets if we only know how to knock, how to give it the necessary blow. The strength and force of the blow come through concentration. There is no limit to the power of the human mind. The more concentrated it is, the more power is brought to bear on one point; that is the secret. (I. 130-31.)

2. The mind takes up various objects, runs into all sorts of things. That is the lower state. There is a higher state of the mind, when it takes up one subject, and excludes all others, of which Samadhi is the result. (I. 273.)

3. The flow of this continuous control of the mind becomes steady when practised day after day, and the mind obtains the faculty of constant concentration. (I. 273.)

4. How are we to know that the mind has become concentrated? Because the idea of time will vanish. The more time passes unnoticed the more concentrated we are. In common life we see that when we are interested in a book we do not note the time at all, and when we leave the

book we are often surprised to find how many hours have passed. All time will have the tendency to come and stand in the one present. So the definition is given, when the past and present come and stand in one, the mind is said to be concentrated. (I. 273-74.)

5. Herein is the difference between man and the animals—man has the greater power of concentration. The difference in their power of concentration also constitutes the difference between man and man. Compare the lowest with the highest man. The difference is in the degree of concentration. This is the only difference. (VI. 37.)

6. Everybody's mind becomes concentrated at times. We all concentrate upon those things we love, and we love those things upon which we concentrate our minds. (V. 37.)

7. We should put our mind on things; they should not draw our minds to them. We are usually forced to concentrate. Our minds are forced to become fixed upon different things by an attraction in them which we cannot resist. To control the mind, to place it just where we want it, requires special training. It cannot be done in any other way. In the study of religion the control of the mind is absolutely necessary. We have to turn the mind back upon itself in this study. (VI. 39.)

8. Concentration of the powers of the mind is our only instrument to help us see God. If you know one soul (your own), you know all souls, past, present and to come. The will concentrates the mind, certain things excite and control this will, such as reason, love, devotion, breathing, etc. The concentrated mind is a lamp that shows us every corner of the soul. (VII. 59-60.)

9. *Q.*—How is it that desires rise even after mental concentration is acquired?

A. —Those are the outcome of previous Samskaras (deep-rooted impressions or tendencies). When Buddha was on the point of merging in Samadhi (superconsciousness), Mara made his appearance. There was really no Mara extraneous to the mind; it was only the external reflection of the mind's previous Samskaras. (VI. 487.)

10. Concentration is the essence of all knowledge; nothing can be done without it. Ninety per cent of thought force is wasted by the ordinary human being, and therefore he is constantly committing blunders; the trained man or mind never makes a mistake. (VI. 123-24.)

11. When the mind is concentrated and turned backward on itself, all within us will be our servants, not our masters.... The Hindu concentrated on the internal world, upon the unseen

realms in the self, and developed the science of Yoga. Yoga is controlling the senses, will, and mind. The benefit of its study is that we learn to control instead of being controlled. Mind seems to be layer on layer. Our real goal is to cross all these intervening strata of our being and find God. (VI. 123-24.)

12. This is what Raja-Yoga proposes to teach. The goal of all its teaching is how to concentrate the mind, then, how to discover the innermost recesses of our own minds, then, how to generalise their contents and form our own conclusions from them. It, therefore, never asks the question what our religion is, whether we are Deists, or Atheists, whether Christians, Jews, or Buddhists. We are human beings; that is sufficient. Every human being has the right and the power to seek for religion. Every human being has the right to ask the reason, and to have his question answered by himself, if he only takes the trouble. (I. 131.)

IX

DUTY

1. The idea of duty varies much among different nations: in one country, if a man does not do certain things, people will say he has acted wrongly; while if he does those very things in another country, people will say that he did not act rightly; and yet we know that there must be some universal idea of duty.... The important thing is to know that there are gradations of duty and of morality—that the duty of one state of life, in one set of circumstances will not and cannot be that of another. (I. 37.)

2. Our first duty is not to hate ourselves; because to advance we must have faith in ourselves first and then in God. He who has no faith in himself can never have faith in God. (I. 38.)

3. To give an objective definition of duty is ...entirely impossible. Yet there is duty from the subjective side. Any action that makes us go Godward is a good action, and is our duty; any action that makes us go downward is evil, and is not our duty. (I. 64.)

4. Every man should take up his own ideal and endeavour to accomplish it; that is a surer way of progress than taking up other men's

ideals, which he can never hope to accomplish. (I. 41.)

5. No man can long occupy satisfactorily a position for which he is not fit. There is no use in grumbling against nature s adjustment. He who does the lower work is not therefore a lower man. No man is to be judged by the mere nature of his duties, but all should be judged by the manner and the spirit in which they perform them. (I. 66.)

6. By doing well the duty which is nearest to us, the duty which is in our hands now, we make ourselves stronger; and improving our strength in this manner step by step, we may even reach a state in which it shall be our privilege to do the most coveted and honoured duties in life and in society. (V. 240.)

7. Every duty is holy, and devotion to duty is the highest form of the worship of God. (V. 240.)

8. We find ourselves in the position for which we are fit, each ball finds its own hole; and if one has some capacity above another, the world will find that out too, in this universal adjusting that goes on. So it is no use to grumble.... What is the use of fighting and complaining? That will not help us to better things. He who grumbles at the little thing that has fallen to his lot to do, will grumble at everything. Always grumbling

DUTY

he will lead a miserable life, and everything will be a failure. But that man who does his duty as he goes, putting his shoulder to the wheel, will see the light, and higher and higher duties will fall to his share. (V. 241-42.)

9. When you are doing any work, do not think of anything beyond. Do it as worship, as the highest worship, and devote your whole life to it for the time being. (I. 71.)

10. It is the worker who is attached to results that grumbles about the nature of the duty which has fallen to his lot; to the unattached worker all duties are equally good, and form efficient instruments with which selfishness and sensuality may be killed, and the freedom of the soul secured. (I. 71.)

11. We are all apt to think too highly of ourselves. Our duties are determined by our deserts to a much larger extent than we are willing to grant. Competition rouses envy, and it kills the kindliness of the heart. To the grumbler all duties are distasteful; nothing will ever satisfy him, and his whole life is doomed to prove a failure. Let us work on, doing as we go whatever happens to be our duty, and being ever ready to put our shoulders to the wheel. Then surely shall we see the Light! (I. 71.)

12. You should cultivate a noble nature by doing your duty. By doing our duty we get rid

of the idea of duty; and then and then only we feel everything as done by God. We are but machines in His hand. This body is opaque, God is the lamp. Whatever is going out of the body is God's. You don't feel it. You feel "I". This is delusion. You must learn calm submission to the will of God. Duty is the best school for it. This duty is morality. Drill yourself to be thoroughly submissive. Get rid of the "I". No humbuggism. Then you can get rid of the idea of duty; for all is His. Then you go on, naturally, forgiving, forgetting, etc. (VI. 118.)

13. Duty is seldom sweet. It is only when love greases its wheels that it runs smoothly; it is a continuous friction otherwise. How else could parents do their duties to their children, husbands to their wives and vice versa? Do we not meet with cases of friction every day in our lives? Duty is sweet only through love. (I. 67.)

14. How easy it is to interpret slavery as duty —the morbid attachment of flesh to flesh as duty! Men go out into the world and struggle and fight for money or for any other thing to which they get attached. Ask them why they do it. They say, "It is a duty." It is the absurd greed for gold and gain, and they try to cover it with a few flowers. (I. 103).

15. Duty becomes a disease with us; it drags us ever forward. It catches hold of us and makes

DUTY

our whole life miserable. It is the bane of human life. This duty, this idea of duty is the midday summer sun which scorches the innermost soul of mankind. Look at those poor slaves to duty! Duty leaves them no time to say prayers, no time to bathe. Duty is ever on them. They go out and work. Duty is on them! They come home and think of the work for the next day. Duty is on them! It is living a slave's life, at last dropping down in the street and dying in harness, like a horse. This is duty as it is understood. The only true duty is to be unattached and to work as free beings, to give up all work unto God. (I. 103.)

X

EDUCATION

1. Education is the manifestation of the perfection already in man. (IV. 358.)

2. What is education? Is it book-learning? No. Is it diverse knowledge? Not even that. The training by which the current and expression of will are brought under control and become fruitful is called education. Now consider, is that education as a result of which the will, being continuously choked by force through generations, is now well-nigh killed out; is that education under whose sway even the old ideas, let alone the new ones, are disappearing one by one; is that education which is slowly making man a machine? (IV. 490.)

3. The true education is not yet conceived of amongst us. I never define anything, still it may be described as a development of faculty, not an accumulation of words, or, as a training of individuals to will rightly and efficiently. (V. 231.)

4. A child teaches itself. But you can *help* it to go forward in its own way. What you can do, is not of the positive nature, but of the negative. You can take away the obstacles, but knowledge comes out of its own nature. Loosen

the soil a little, so that it may come out easily. Put a hedge round it; see that it is not killed by anything, and there your work stops. You cannot do anything else. The rest is manifestation from *within* its own nature. So with the education of a child. A child educates itself. You come to hear me, and when you go home, compare what you have learnt, and you will find you have thought out the same thing; I have only given it expression. I can never teach you anything; you will have to teach yourself, but I can help you perhaps in giving expression to that thought. (IV. 55.)

5. You see, no one can teach anybody. The teacher spoils everything by thinking that he is teaching. Thus Vedanta says that within man is all knowledge—even in a boy it is so—and it requires only an awakening, and that much is the work of a teacher. We have to do only so much for the boys that they may learn to apply their own intellect to the proper use of their hands, legs, ears, eyes, etc., and finally everything will become easy. (V. 366.)

6. Haven't you read the stories from the Upanishads? I will tell you one. Satyakama went to live the life of a Brahmacharin with his Guru. The Guru gave into his charge some cows and sent him away to the forest with them. Many months passed by, and when Satyakama saw

that the number of cows was doubled, he thought of returning to his Guru. On his way back, one of the bulls, the fire, and some other animals gave him instruction about the Highest Brahman. When the disciple came back, the Guru at once saw by a mere glance at his face that the disciple had learnt the knowledge of the Supreme Brahman. Now, the moral this story is meant to teach is that true education is gained by living in constant communion with Nature. (V. 369.)

7. To me the very essence of education is concentration of mind, not the collecting of facts. If I had to do my education over again, and had any voice in the matter, I would not study facts at all. I would develop the power of concentration and detachment, and then with a perfect instrument I could collect facts at will. Side by side, in the child, should be developed the power of concentration and detachment. (VI. 38-39.)

8. Well, you consider a man as educated if only he can pass some examinations and deliver good lectures. The education which does not help the common mass of people to equip themselves for the struggle for life, which does not bring out strength of character, a spirit of philanthropy, and the courage of a lion—is it worth the name? Real education is that which enables one to stand on his own legs. The education

EDUCATION

that you are receiving now in schools and colleges is only making you a race of dyspeptics. You are working like machines merely, and living a jelly-fish existence. (VII. 147-48.)

9. Education is not the amount of information that is put into your brain and runs riot there, undigested all your life. We must have life-building, man-making, character-making, assimilation of ideas. If you have assimilated five ideas and made them your life and character, you have more education than any man who has got by heart a whole library. If education were identical with information, the libraries would be the greatest sages in the world and encyclopaedias the Rishis. (III. 302.)

10. Negative thoughts weaken men. Do you not find that where parents are constantly taxing their sons to read and write, telling them they will never learn anything, and calling them fools and so forth, the latter do actually turn out to be so in many cases? If you speak kind words to boys and encourage them, they are bound to improve in time. What holds good of children, also holds good of children in the region of higher thoughts. If you can give them positive ideas, people will grow up to be men and learn to stand on their own legs. (VII. 170.)

11. In language and literature, in poetry and in arts, in everything we must point out not

the mistakes that people are making in their thoughts and actions, but the way in which they will gradually be able to do these things better. Pointing out mistakes wounds a man's feelings. We have seen how Sri Ramakrishna would encourage even those whom we considered as worthless, and change the very course of their lives thereby! His very method of teaching was a unique phenomenon. (VII. 170-71.)

12. Knowledge is inherent in man; no knowledge comes from outside; it is all inside. What we say a man "knows", should, in strict psychological language, be what he "discovers" or "unveils"; what a man "learns" is really what he "discovers", by taking the cover off his own soul, which is a mine of infinite knowledge. We say Newton discovered gravitation. Was it sitting anywhere in a corner waiting for him? It was in his own mind; the time came and he found it out. (I. 28.)

13. All knowledge that the world has ever received comes from the mind; the infinite library of the universe is in your own mind. The external world is simply the suggestion, the occasion, which sets you to study your own mind, but the object of your study is always your own mind. The falling of an apple gave the suggestion to Newton, and he studied his own mind; he re-arranged all the previous links of thought

in his mind and discovered a new link among them, which we call the law of gravitation. It was not in the apple nor in anything in the centre of the earth. (I. 28.)

14. All knowledge, secular or spiritual, is in the human mind. In many cases it is not discovered, but remains covered, and when the covering is being slowly taken off we say "we are learning", and the advance of knowledge is made by the advance of this process of uncovering. The man from whom this veil is being lifted is the more knowing man; the man upon whom it lies thick is ignorant, and the man from whom it has entirely gone is all-knowing, omniscient. (I. 28.)

15. Like fire in a piece of flint, knowledge exists in the mind; suggestion is the friction which brings it out. (I. 28.)

16. No one was ever really taught by another; each of us has to teach himself. The external teacher offers only the suggestion which rouses the internal teacher to work to understand things. (I. 93.)

17. Education is not filling the mind with a lot of facts. Perfecting the instrument and getting complete mastery of my own mind [is the ideal of education]. If I want to concentrate my mind upon a point, it goes there, and the moment I call, it is free [again]. (I. 510.)

XI

ETHICS

1. *That society is the greatest, where the highest truths become practical.* That is my opinion, and if society is not fit for the highest truths, make it so, and the sooner, the better. Stand up, men and women, in this spirit, dare to believe in the Truth, dare to practise the Truth! (II. 85.)

2. Who knows which is the truer ideal? The apparent power and strength, as held in the West, or the fortitude in suffering, of the East?

The West says: "We minimise evil by conquering it." India says: "We destroy evil by suffering, until evil is nothing to us, it becomes positive enjoyment." Well, both are great ideals. Who knows which will survive in the long run? Who knows which attitude will really most benefit humanity? Who knows which will disarm and conquer animality? Will it be suffering, or doing?

In the meantime, let us not destroy each other's ideals. We are both intent upon the same work, which is the annihilation of evil. You take up your method; let us take up our method. Let us not destroy the ideal. I do not say to the West: "Take up our method." Certainly not.

The goal is the same, but the methods can never be the same. And so, after hearing about the ideals of India, I hope that you will say in the same breath to India: "We know the goal, the ideal, is all right for us both. You follow your own ideal. You follow your method in your own way, and God speed you!" My message in life is to ask the East and West not to quarrel over different ideals, but to show them that the goal is the same in both cases, however opposite it may appear. As we wend our way through this mazy vale of life, let us bid each other Godspeed. (IV. 76-77.)

3. The work of ethics has been, and will be in the future, not the destruction of variation and the establishment of sameness in the external world, which is impossible, for it would bring death and annihilation—but to recognise the unity in spite of all these variations, to recognise the God within, in spite of everything that frightens us, to recognise that infinite strength as the property of everyone in spite of all apparent weakness, and to recognise the eternal, infinite, essential purity of the soul in spite of everything to the contrary that appears on the surface. (I. 436.)

4. Coming to ethics, we find a tremendous departure. It is, perhaps, the only science which makes a bold departure from this fight. For

ethics is unity; its basis is love. It will not look at this variation. The one aim of ethics is this unity, this sameness. The highest ethical codes that mankind has discovered up to the present time, know no variation, they have no time to stop to look into it; their one end is to make for that sameness. The Indian mind, being more analytical—I mean the Vedantic mind—found this unity as the result of all its analysis, and wanted to base everything upon this one idea of unity. (I. 432.)

5. Karma-Yoga, therefore, is a system of ethics and religion intended to attain freedom through unselfishness, and by good works. The Karma-Yogi need not believe in any doctrine whatever. He may not believe even in God, may not ask what his soul is, not think of any metaphysical speculation. He has got his own special aim of realising selflessness; and he has to work it out himself. Every moment of his life must be realisation because he has to solve by mere work, without the help of doctrine or theory, the very same problem to which the Jnani applies his reason and inspiration and the Bhakta his love. (I. 111.)

6. In modern times this millennial aspiration takes the form of equality—of liberty, equality and fraternity. This is also fanaticism. True equality has never been and never can be on

earth. How can we all be equal here? This impossible kind of equality implies total death. (I. 113.)

7. Yet this idea of realising the millennium is a great motive power. Just as inequality is necessary for creation itself, so the struggle to limit it is also necessary. If there were no struggle to become free and get back to God, there would be no creation either. It is the difference between these two forces that determines the nature of the motives of men. There will always be these motives to work, some tending towards bondage and others towards freedom. (I. 115.)

8. That some will be stronger physically than others, and will thus naturally be able to subdue or defeat the weak, is a self-evident fact, but that because of this strength they should gather unto themselves all the attainable happiness of this life, is not according to law, and the fight has been against it. That some people through natural aptitude, should be able to accumulate more wealth than others, is natural; but that on account of this power to acquire wealth they should tyrannise and ride roughshod over those who cannot acquire so much wealth, is not a part of the law, and the fight has been against that. The enjoyment of advantage over another is privilege, and throughout ages, the aim of morality has been its destruction. This is the

work which tends towards sameness, towards unity, without destroying variety. (I. 435.)

9. Change is always subjective. All through evolution you find that the conquest of nature comes by change in the subject. Apply this to religion and morality, and you will find that the conquest of evil comes by the change in the subjective alone. That is how the Advaita system gets its whole force, on the subjective side of man. To talk of evil and misery is nonsense, because they do not exist outside. If I am immune against all anger, I never feel angry. If I am proof against all hatred, I never feel hatred. (II. 137-38.)

10. Good and evil are only a question of degree: more manifested or less manifested. Just take the example of our own lives. How many things we see in our childhood which we think to be good, but which really are evil, and how many things seem to be evil which are good! How the ideas change! How an idea goes up and up! What we thought very good at one time we do not think so good now. So good and evil are but superstitions, and do not exist. The difference is only in degree. It is all a manifestation of that Atman; He is being manifested in everything; only, when the manifestation is very thick we call it evil; and when it is very thin, we call it good. (II. 420.)

11. Ethics always says, "Not I, but thou." Its motto is, "Not self, but non-self." The vain ideas of individualism to which man clings when he is trying to find that Infinite Power, or that Infinite Pleasure through the senses, have to be given up, say the laws of ethics. You have to put *yourself* last, and others before you. The senses say, "Myself first." Ethics says, "I must hold myself last." Thus, all codes of ethics are based upon this renunciation; destruction, not construction, of the individual on the material plane. That Infinite will never find expression upon the material plane, nor is it possible or thinkable. (II. 62-63.)

12. The great error in all ethical systems, without exception, has been the failure of teaching the means by which man could refrain from doing evil. All the systems of ethics teach, "Do not steal!" Very good; but why does a man steal? Because all stealing, robbing, and other evil actions, as a rule, have become automatic. The systematic robber, thief, liar, unjust man and woman, are all these in spite of themselves! It is really a tremendous psychological problem. We should look upon man in the most charitable light. It is not so easy to be good. What are you but mere machines until you are free? Should you be proud because you are good? Certainly not. You are good because you cannot help it. Another is bad because he cannot help

it. If you were in his position, who knows what you would have been? The woman in the street, or the thief in the jail, is the Christ that is being sacrificed that you may be a good man. Such is the law of balance. All the thieves and the murderers, all the unjust, the weakest, the wickedest, the devils, they all are my Christ! I owe a worship to the God Christ and to the demon Christ! That is my doctrine, I cannot help it. My salutation goes to the feet of the good, the saintly, and to the feet of the wicked and the devilish! They are all my teachers, all are my spiritual fathers, all are my Saviours. I may curse one and yet benefit by his failings; I may bless another and benefit by his good deeds. This is as true as that I stand here. I have to sneer at the woman walking in the street, because society wants it! She, my Saviour, she, whose street-walking is the cause of the chastity of other women! Think of that. Think, men and women, of this question in your mind. It is a truth—a bare, bold truth! As I see more of the world, see more of men and women, this conviction grows stronger. Whom shall I blame? Whom shall I praise? Both sides of the shield must be seen. (II. 33-34.)

XII

FAITH

1. All such ideas as we can do this, or cannot do that are superstitions. We can do everything. The Vedanta teaches men to have faith in themselves first. As certain religions of the world say that a man who does not believe in a Personal God outside of himself is an atheist, so the Vedanta says, a man who does not believe in himself is an atheist. Not believing in the glory of our own soul is what the Vedanta calls atheism. (II. 294.)

2. The ideal of faith in ourselves is of the greatest help to us. If faith in ourselves had been more extensively taught and practised, I am sure a very large portion of the evils and miseries that we have, would have vanished. Throughout the history of mankind, if any motive power has been more potent than another in the lives of all great men and women, it is that of faith in themselves. Born with the consciousness that they were to be great, they became great. (II. 301.)

3. Let a man go down as low as possible; there must come a time when out of sheer desperation he will take an upward curve and will learn to have faith in himself. But it is better

for us that we should know it from the very first. Why should we have all these bitter experiences in order to gain faith in ourselves? (II. 301.)

4. We can see that all the difference between man and man is owing to the existence or non-existence of faith in himself. Faith in ourselves will do everything. I have experienced it in my own life, and am still doing so, and as I grow older that faith is becoming stronger and stronger. He is an atheist who does not believe in himself. The old religions said that he was an atheist who did not believe in God. The new religion says that he is an atheist who does not believe in himself. But it is not selfish faith, because the Vedanta, again, is the doctrine of Oneness. It means faith in all, because you are all. (II. 301.)

5. It is the great faith which will make the world better. I am sure of that. He is the highest man who can say with truth, "I know all about myself". Do you know how much energy, how many powers, how many forces, are still lurking behind that frame of yours? What scientist has known all that is in man? Millions of years have passed since man came here, and yet but one infinitesimal part of his powers has been manifested. Therefore, you must not say that you are weak. How do you know what possibilities lie behind that degradation on the surface? You

know but little of that which is within you. For behind you is the ocean of infinite power and blessedness. (II. 301-02.)

6. Faith, faith, faith in ourselves, faith, faith in God—this is the secret of greatness. If you have faith in all the three hundred and thirty millions of your mythological gods, and in all the Gods which foreigners have now and again introduced into your midst, and still have no faith in yourselves, there is no salvation for you. Have faith in yourselves, and stand up on that faith and be strong; that is what we need. (III. 190.)

7. We have lost faith in ourselves. Therefore, to preach the Advaita aspect of the Vedanta is necessary to rouse up the hearts of men, to show them the glory of their souls. It is therefore that I preach this Advaita, and I do so not as a sectarian, but upon universal and widely acceptable grounds. (III. 191.)

8. Whether dualistic, qualified monistic, or monistic, they all firmly believe that everything is in the soul itself; it has only to come out and manifest itself. Therefore, this Shraddha is what I want, and what all of us here want, this faith in ourselves, and before you is the great task to get that faith. Give up the awful disease that is creeping into our national blood, that idea of ridiculing everything, that loss of seriousness.

Give that up. Be strong and have this Shraddha, and everything else is bound to follow. (III. 320.)

9. Be not afraid of anything. You will do marvellous work. The moment you fear, you are nobody. It is fear that is the great cause of misery in the world. It is fear that is the greatest of all superstitions. It is fear that is the cause of our woes, and it is fearlessness that brings heaven even in a moment. Therefore, "Arise, awake, and stop not till the goal is reached". (III. 320-21.)

10. If a man, day and night, thinks he is miserable, low and nothing, nothing he becomes. If you say yea, yea, "I am, I am", so shall you be; and if you say "I am not", think that you are not, and day and night meditate upon the fact that you are nothing, aye, nothing shall you be. That is the great fact which you ought to remember. We are the children of the Almighty, we are the sparks of the infinite, divine fire. How can you be nothings? We are everything, ready to do everything, we can do everything, and man must do everything. (III. 376.)

11. This faith in themselves was in the hearts of our ancestors, this faith in themselves was the motive power that pushed them forward and forward in the march of civilisation, and if there has been degeneration, if there has been defect, mark my words, you will find that degradation

FAITH

to have started on the day our people lost faith in themselves. (III. 376.)

12. Losing faith in one's self means losing faith in God. Do you believe in that Infinite, good Providence working in and through you? If you believe that this Omnipresent One is present in every atom, is through and through, Ota-Prota, as the Sanskrit word goes, penetrating your body, mind, and soul, how can you lose heart? (III. 376.)

XIII

FOOD

1. We have to take care what sort of food we eat at the beginning, and when we have got strength enough, when our practice is well advanced, we need not be so careful in this respect. While the plant is growing it must be hedged round, lest it be injured, but when it becomes a tree the hedges are taken away; it is strong enough to withstand all assaults. (I. 136.)

2. Certain regulations as to food are necessary; we must use the food which brings the purest mind. (I. 136.)

3. There are certain kinds of food that produce a certain change in the mind; we see it every day. There are other sorts which produce a change in the body, and in the long run have a tremendous effect on the mind. It is a great thing to learn; a good deal of the misery we suffer is occasioned by the food we take. You find that after a heavy and indigestible meal it is very hard to control the mind; it is running, running all the time. There are certain foods which are exciting; if you eat such food, you find that you cannot control the mind. (IV. 4.)

4. Are we to pass our lives discussing all the time about the purity and impurity of food only,

or are we to practise the restraining of our senses? Surely, the restraining of the senses is the main object; and the discrimination of good and bad, pure and impure food, only helps one, to a certain extent, in getting that end. (V. 403-04.)

5. There are according to our scriptures, three things which make food impure: (1) Jati-dosha, or natural defects of a certain class of food, like onions, garlic, etc.; (2) Nimitta-dosha, or defects arising from the presence of external impurities in it, such as dead insects, dust, etc., that attach to sweetmeats bought from shops; (3) Ashraya-dosha, or defects that arise by the food coming from evil sources, as when it has been touched and handled by wicked persons. Special care should be taken to avoid the first and second classes of defects. But in this country men pay no regard to these very two, and go on fighting for the third alone, the very one that none but a Yogi could really discriminate! (V. 404.)

6. The beginner must pay particular attention to all such dietetic rules as have come down from the line of his accredited teachers; but the extravagant, meaningless fanaticism, which has driven religion entirely to the kitchen, as may be noticed in the case of many of our sects, without any hope of the noble truth of that religion ever coming out to the sunlight of spirituality, is a

peculiar sort of pure and simple materialism. (III. 66.)

7. You speak of the meat-eating Kshatriya; meat or no meat, it is they who are the fathers of all that is noble and beautiful in Hinduism. Who wrote the Upanishads? Who was Rama? Who was Krishna? Who was Buddha? Who were the Tirthankaras of the Jains?... Is God a nervous fool like you that the flow of His river of mercy would be dammed up by a piece of meat? If such be He, His value is not a pie! (IV. 359.)

8. The taking of life is undoubtedly sinful. But so long as vegetable food is not made suitable to the human system, through progress in Chemistry, there is no alternative but meat-eating. So long as man shall have to live a Rajasika (active) life under circumstances like the present, there is no other way except through meat-eating. It is true that the Emperor Asoka saved the lives of millions of animals by the threat of the sword, but, is not the slavery of a thousand years more dreadful than that? Taking the life of a few goats against the inability to protect the honour of one's wife and daughter, and to save the morsels for one's children from robbing hands—which of these is more sinful? Rather let those belonging to the upper ten, who do not earn their livelihood by manual labour,

not take meat; but the forcing of vegetarianism upon those who have to earn their bread by labouring day and night, is one of the causes of the loss of our national freedom. (IV. 486-87.)

9. More than ninety per cent of those whom you now take to be men with the Sattva quality are only steeped in the deepest Tamas. Enough if you find one-sixteenth of them to be really Sattvika? What we want now is an immense awakening of Rajasika energy, for the whole country is wrapped in the shroud of Tamas. The people of this land must be fed and clothed— must be awakened—must be made more fully active. Otherwise they will become inert, as inert as trees and stones. So, I say, eat large quantities of fish and meat, my boy! (V. 402-03.)

10. To eat meat is surely barbarous and vegetable food is certainly purer—who can deny that? For him surely is a strict vegetarian diet, whose one end is to lead solely a spiritual life. But he who has to steer the boat of his life with strenuous labour through the constant life-and-death struggles and the competition of this world, must of necessity take meat. So long as there will be in human society such a thing as the triumph of the strong over the weak, animal food is required, or some other suitable substitute for it has to be discovered; otherwise, the weak will naturally be crushed under the feet of the strong.

It will not do to quote solitary instances of the good effect of vegetable food on some particular person or persons; compare one nation with another, and then draw conclusions. (V. 485.)

XIV

FREEDOM AND MUKTI (Salvation)

1. The mind cannot be easily conquered. Minds that rise into waves at the approach of every little thing, at the slightest provocation or danger, in what a state they must be! What to talk of greatness or spirituality, when these changes come over the mind? This unstable condition of the mind must be changed. We must ask ourselves how far we can be acted upon by the external world, and how far we can stand on our own feet in spite of all the forces outside us. When we have succeeded in preventing all the forces in the world from throwing us off our balance, then alone we have attained to freedom, and not before. That is salvation. (I. 426.)

2. Everything that we perceive around us is struggling towards freedom, from the atom to the man, from insentient, lifeless particle of matter to the highest existence on earth, the human soul. The whole universe is in fact the result of this struggle for freedom. (I. 108.)

3. All that we see in the universe has for its basis this one struggle towards freedom; it is under the impulse of this tendency that the saint prays and the robber robs. When the line of

action is not a proper one we call it evil, and when the manifestation of it is proper and high we call it good. But the impulse is the same, the struggle towards freedom. (I. 108-09.)

4. Freedom is the one goal of nature, sentient or insentient; and consciously or unconsciously everything is struggling towards that goal. The freedom which the saint seeks is very different from that which the robber seeks; the freedom loved by the saint leads him to the enjoyment of infinite, unspeakable bliss, while that on which the robber has set his heart only forges other bonds for his soul. (I. 109.)

5. We say that it is freedom that we are to seek, and that that freedom is God. It is the same happiness as in everything else; but when man seeks it in something which is finite, he gets only a spark of it. The thief when he steals gets the same happiness as the man who finds it in God; but the thief gets only a spark with a mass of misery. The real happiness is God. Love is God, freedom is God; and everything that is bondage is not God. (V. 288.)

6. Man has freedom already, but he will have to discover it. He has it but every moment he forgets it. That discovering, consciously or unconsciously, is the whole life of every one. But the difference between the sage and the ignorant

man is that one does it consciously and the other unconsciously. (V. 288.)

7. The idea of freedom is the only true idea of salvation—freedom from everything, the senses, whether of pleasure or pain, from good as well as evil.

More than this even. We must be free from death; and to be free from death, we must be free from life. Life is but a dream of death. Where there is life, there will be death; so get away from life if you would be rid of death. (VI. 93.)

8. We are ever free if we would believe it, only have faith enough. You are the soul, free and eternal, ever free, ever blessed. Have faith enough and you will be free in a minute.

Everything in time, space, and causation is bound. The soul is beyond all time, all space, all causation. That which is bound is nature, not the soul.

Therefore proclaim your freedom and be what you are—ever free, ever blessed. (VI. 93.)

9. To acquire freedom we have to go beyond the limitations of this universe; it cannot be found here. Perfect equilibrium, or what the Christians call the peace that passeth understanding, cannot be had in this universe, nor in heaven, nor in any place where our mind and thoughts can go, where the senses can feel, or

which the imagination can conceive. No such place can give us the freedom, because all such places would be within our universe, and it is limited by space, time, and causation. (I. 97.)

10. If we give up our attachment to this little universe of the senses or of the mind, we shall be free immediately. The only way to come out of bondage is to go beyond the limitations of law, to go beyond causation. (I. 98.)

11. Blessedness, eternal peace arising from perfect freedom, is the highest conception of religion, underlying all the ideas of God in Vedanta—absolutely free Existence, not bound by anything, no change, no nature, nothing that can produce a change in Him. This same freedom is in you and in me and is the only real freedom. (I. 337.)

12. Worship of God, worship of the holy ones, concentration and meditation and unselfish work, these are the ways of breaking away from Maya's net; but we must first have the strong desire to get free. The flash of light that will illumine the darkness for us is in us; it is the knowledge that is our nature (there is no "birthright", we were never born). All that we have to do is to drive away the clouds that cover it. (VII. 92.)

13. There is to be found in every religion the manifestation of this struggle towards freedom.

It is the groundwork of all morality, of unselfishness, which means getting rid of the idea that men are the same as their little body. When we see a man doing good work, helping others, it means that he cannot be confined within the limited circle of "me and mine". There is no limit to this getting out of selfishness. All the great systems of ethics preach absolute unselfishness as the goal. Supposing this absolute unselfishness can be reached by a man, what becomes of him? He is no more the little Mr. So-and-so; he has acquired infinite expansion. That little personality which he had before is now lost to him for ever; he has become infinite, and the attainment of this infinite expansion is indeed the goal of all religions and of all moral and philosophical teachings. (I. 109.)

14. To be more free is the goal of all our efforts, for only in perfect freedom can there be perfection. This effort to attain freedom underlies all forms of worship, whether we know it or not. (I. 333.)

15. Freedom is the motive of the universe, freedom its goal. The laws of nature are the methods through which we are struggling to reach that freedom under the guidance of Mother. This universal struggle for freedom attains its highest expression in man in the conscious desire to be free.

This freedom is attained by the threefold means of work, worship, and knowledge.

     (a) Work—constant, unceasing effort to help others and love others.

     (b) Worship—consists in prayer, praise and meditation.

     (c) Knowledge—that follows meditation. (V. 434.)

16. We find by analysis on philosophic grounds that we are not free. But there will remain this factor, this consciousness that I am free. What we have to explain is, how that comes. We will find that we have these two impulsions in us. Our reason tells us that all our actions are caused, and at the same time, with every impulse we are asserting our freedom. The solution of the Vedanta is that there is freedom inside—that the soul is really free—but that the soul's actions are percolating through body and mind, which are not free. (V. 290.)

17. All nature is bound by law, the law of its own action; and this law can never be broken. If you could break a law of nature, all nature would come to an end in an instant. There would be no more nature. He who attains freedom breaks the law of nature, and for him nature fades away and has no more power over him. Each one will break the law but once and for

ever, and that will end his trouble with nature. (VI. 99-100.)

18. The whole object of their system is by constant struggle to become perfect, to become divine, to reach God and see God, and this reaching God, seeing God, becoming perfect even as the Father in heaven is perfect, constitutes the religion of the Hindus.

And what becomes of a man when he attains perfection? He lives a life of bliss infinite. He enjoys infinite and perfect bliss having obtained the only thing in which man ought to have pleasure, namely God, and enjoys the bliss with God. (I. 13.)

19. We must remember that our religion lays down distinctly and clearly, that every one who wants salvation must pass through the stage of Rishihood—must become a Mantra-drashta, must see God. That is salvation; that is the law laid down by our Scriptures. (III. 284.)

20. Isolation of the soul from all objects, mental and physical, is the goal; when that is attained, the soul will find that it was alone all the time, and it required no one to make it happy. As long as we require someone else to make us happy we are slaves. When the Purusha finds that It is free, and does not require anything to complete Itself, that this Nature is quite

unnecessary, then freedom (Kaivalya) is attained. (V. 239.)

21. The Vedanta teaches that Nirvana can be attained here and now, that we do not have to wait for death to reach it. Nirvana is the realisation of the Self; and after having once known that, if only for an instant, never again can one be deluded by the mirage of the personality. Having eyes, we must see the apparent, but all the time we know what it is; we have found out its true nature. It is the screen that hides the Self, which is unchanging. The screen opens, and we find the Self behind it. All change is in the screen. In the saint the screen is thin, and the reality can almost shine through. In the sinner the screen is thick, and we are liable to lose sight of the truth that the Atman is there, as well as behind the saint's screen. When the screen is wholly removed, we find it really never existed—that we were the Atman and nothing else, even the screen is forgotten. (V. 284-85.)

22. It is not that when a man becomes free, he will stop and become a dead lump; but he will be more active than any other being, because every other being acts only under compulsion, he alone through freedom. (V. 286.)

23. Ignorance is death, knowledge is life. (I. 52.)

24. Liberation means entire freedom—freedom

from the bondage of good, as well as from the bondage of evil. A golden chain is as much a chain as an iron one. (I. 55.)

25. You must retain great strength in your mind and words. "I am low, I am low," repeating these ideas in the mind man belittles and degrades himself. Therefore the Shastras say,

मुक्ताभिमानी मुक्तोहि बद्धो बद्धाभिमान्यपि ।
किं वदन्तीह सत्येयं या मतिः सा गतिर्भवेत् ॥

"He who thinks himself free, free he becomes; he who thinks himself bound, bound he remains" —this popular saying "As one thinks, so one becomes" is true. He alone who is always awake to the idea of freedom, becomes free; he who thinks he is bound, endures life after life in the state of bondage. (VII. 135.)

26. Salvation means knowing the truth. We do not become anything; we are what we are. Salvation [comes] by faith and not by work. It is a question of *knowledge*! You must *know* what you are, and it is done. (I. 512.)

XV

GITA

1. The greatness of little things, that is what the Gita teaches, bless the old book! (VI. 436.)

2. This is the one central idea in the Gita: Work incessantly, but be not attached to it. (I. 53.)

3. The Bhagavad-Gita is the best commentary we have on the Vedanta philosophy—curiously enough the scene is laid on the battlefield, where Krishna teaches this philosophy to Arjuna, and the doctrine which stands out luminously in every page of the Gita is intense activity, but in the midst of it, eternal calmness. This is the secret of work, to attain which is the goal of the Vedanta. (II. 292.)

4. We are reading the Gita by candle-light, but numbers of insects are being burnt to death. Thus it is seen that some evil clings to work. Those who work without any consciousness of their lower ego are not affected with evil, for they work for the good of the world. To work without motive, to work unattached, brings the highest bliss and freedom. This secret of Karma-Yoga is taught by the Lord Sri Krishna in the Gita. (V. 249.)

5. In reading the Bhagavad-Gita many of you

in Western countries may have felt astonished in the second chapter, wherein Sri Krishna calls Arjuna a hypocrite and a coward because of his refusal to fight, or offer resistance, on account of his adversaries being his friends and relatives, making the plea that non-resistance was the highest ideal of love. This is a great lesson for us all to learn, that in all matters the two extremes are alike; the extreme positive and the extreme negative are always similar.... Arjuna became a coward at the sight of the mighty array against him; his "love" made him forget his duty towards his country and king. This is why Sri Krishna told him that he was a hypocrite: Thou talkest like a wise man, but thy actions betray thee to be a coward; therefore stand up and fight! (I. 38-39.)

6. We read in the Bhagavad-Gita again and again that we must all work incessantly. All work is by nature composed of good and evil. We cannot do any work which will not do some good somewhere; there cannot be any work which will not cause some harm somewhere. Every work must necessarily be a mixture of good and evil; yet we are commanded to work incessantly. Good and evil will both have their results, will produce their Karma. Good action will entail upon us good effect; bad action, bad. But good and bad are both bondages of the soul. The

solution reached in the Gita in regard to this bondage-producing nature of work is that if we do not attach ourselves to the work we do, it will not have any binding effect on our soul. (I. 53.)

7. This is the one cause of misery: we are attached; we are being caught. Therefore says the Gita: Work constantly; work, but be not attached; be not caught. Reserve unto yourself the power of detaching yourself from everything, however beloved, however much the soul might yearn for it, however great the pangs of misery you feel if you are going to leave it; still, reserve the power of leaving it whenever you want. (II. 2-3.)

8. The heart's love is due to only One. To whom? To Him who never changeth.... So says Sri Krishna in the Gita: The Lord is the only one who never changes. His love never fails. Wherever we are and whatever we do, He is ever and ever the same merciful, the same loving heart. He never changes.... We must love Him, and everyone that lives—only in and through Him. This is the keynote. (IV. 128-29.)

9. Gita teaches Karma-Yoga, we should work through Yoga (concentration). In such concentration in action (Karma-Yoga), there is no consciousness of the lower ego present. The consciousness that I am doing this and that is

never present when one works through Yoga. The Western people do not understand this. They say that if there be no consciousness of ego, if this ego is gone, how then can a man work? But when one works with concentration, losing all consciousness of oneself, the work that is done will be infinitely better, and this every one may have experienced in his own life.... The Gita teaches that all works should be done thus. He who is one with the Lord through Yoga performs all his works by becoming immersed in concentration, and does not seek any personal benefit. Such a performance of work brings only good to the world, no evil can come out of it. Those who work thus never do anything for themselves. (V. 247-48.)

10. Aye, if there is anything in the Gita that I like, it is the two verses, coming out strong as the very gist, the very essence, of Krishna's teaching: "He who sees the Supreme Lord dwelling alike in all beings, the Imperishable in things that perish, he sees indeed. For seeing the Lord as the same, everywhere present, he does not destroy the Self by the self, and thus he goes to the highest goal." (III. 193-94.)

11. The Bhagavad-Gita is the best authority on Vedanta. (VII. 57.)

12. Wherein lies the originality of the Gita, which distinguishes it from all preceding Scrip-

tures? It is this: Though before its advent, Yoga, Jnana, Bhakti, etc. had each its strong adherents, they all quarrelled among themselves, each claiming superiority for his own chosen path; no one ever tried to seek for reconciliation among these different paths. It was the author of the Gita who for the first time tried to harmonise these. He took the best from what all the sects then existing had to offer, and threaded them in the Gita. (IV. 106-7.)

13. The reconciliation of the different paths of Dharma, and work without desire or attachment—these are the two special characteristics of the Gita. (IV. 107.)

14. If one reads this one Shloka—(Yield not to unmanliness, O son of Pritha! Ill doth it become thee. Cast off this mean faint-heartedness and arise, O scorcher of thy enemies!)—he gets all the merits of reading the entire Gita; for in this one Shloka lies imbedded the whole message of the Gita. (IV. 110.)

15. Many are of opinion that the Gita was not written at the time of the Mahabharata, but was subsequently added to it. This is not correct. The special teachings of the Gita are to be found in every part of the Mahabharata; and if the Gita is to be expunged, as forming no part of it, every other portion of it which embodies the same teachings should be similarly treated. (V. 247.)

16. The teachings of Krishna as taught by the Gita are the grandest the world has ever known. He who wrote that wonderful poem was one of those rare souls whose lives send a wave of regeneration through the world. The human race will never again see such a brain as his who wrote the Gita. (VII. 22.)

17. This great poem is held to be the crown jewel of all Indian literature. It is a kind of commentary on the Vedas. It shows us that our battle for spirituality must be fought out in this life; so we must not flee from it, but rather compel it to give us all that it holds. As the Gita typifies this struggle for higher things, it is highly poetical to lay the scene in a battlefield. Krishna in the guise of a charioteer to Arjuna, leader of one of the opposing armies, urges him not to be sorrowful, not to fear death, since he knows he is immortal, that nothing which changes can be in the *real* nature of man. Through chapter after chapter, Krishna teaches the higher truths of philosophy and religion to Arjuna. It is these teachings which make this poem so wonderful; practically the whole of the Vedanta philosophy is included in them. (VIII. 8-9.)

XVI

GOD

1. The Hindu does not want to live upon words and theories. If there are existences beyond the ordinary sensuous existence, he wants to come face to face with them. If there is a soul in him which is not matter, if there is an all-merciful universal soul, he will go to Him direct. He must see Him, and that alone can destroy all doubts. So the best proof a Hindu sage gives about the soul, about God, is—"I have seen the soul; I have seen God." (I. 13.)

2. Remember the words of Christ—"Ask, and it shall be given you; seek, and ye shall find; knock, and it shall be opened unto you." These words are literally true, not figures or fiction. They were the outflow of the heart's blood of one of the greatest sons of God, who have ever come to this world of ours; words which came as the fruit of realisation, from a man who had felt and realised God Himself; who had spoken with God, lived with God, a hundred times more intensely, than you or I see this building. (II. 44.)

3. If conformity is the law of the universe, every part of the universe must have been built on the same plan as the whole. So we naturally think that behind the gross material form which

we call this universe of ours, there must be a universe of finer matter, which we call thought, and behind that there must be a Soul, which makes all this thought possible, which commands, which is the enthroned king of this universe. That soul which is behind each mind and each body is called "Pratyagatman", the individual Atman, and that Soul which is behind the universe as its guide, ruler and governor, is God. (II. 425.)

4. Whatever may be the position of Philosophy, whatever may be the position of Metaphysics, so long as there is such a thing as death in the world, so long as there is such a thing as weakness in the human heart, so long as there is a cry going out of the heart of man in his very weakness, there shall be a faith in God. (I. 22.)

5. The child rebels against law as soon as it is born. Its first utterance is a cry, a protest against the bondage in which it finds itself. This longing for freedom produces the idea of a Being who is absolutely free. The concept of God is a fundamental element in the human constitution. In the Vedanta, Sat-chit-ananda (Existence-Knowledge-Bliss) is the highest concept of God possible to the mind. It is the essence of knowledge and is by its nature the essence of bliss. (I. 334.)

6. From Whom all beings are projected, in Whom all live, and unto Whom they all return; that is God. (I. 416.)

7. The whole of Nature is worship of God. Wherever there is life, there is this search for freedom and that freedom is the same as God. (I. 337.)

8. We go through the world like a man pursued by a policeman and see the barest glimpses of the beauty of it. All this fear that pursues us comes from believing in matter. Matter gets its whole existence from the presence of mind behind it. What we see is God percolating through Nature. (VII. 6.)

9. God is still established upon His own majestic changeless Self. You and I try to be one with Him, but plant ourselves upon Nature, upon the trifles of daily life, on money, on fame, on human love and all these changing forms in Nature which make for bondage. (I. 337.)

10. When Nature shines, upon what depends the shining? Upon God and not upon the sun nor the moon nor the stars. Wherever anything shines, whether it is the light in the sun or in our own consciousness, it is He. He shining, all shines after Him. (I. 337.)

11. After so much austerity I have understood this as the real truth—God is present in every

Jiva; there is no other God besides that. "Who serves Jiva, serves God indeed." (VII. 247.)

12. All beings, great or small, are equally manifestations of God; the difference is only in the manifestation. (I. 424.)

13. The sum total of this whole universe is God Himself. Is God then matter? No, certainly not, for matter is that God perceived by the five senses; that God as perceived by the intellect is mind; and when the spirit sees, He is seen as spirit. He is not matter, but whatever is real in matter is He. (I. 375.)

14. There are two ideas of God in our Scriptures; the one the personal, and the other the impersonal. The idea of the Personal God is that He is the omnipresent creator, preserver and destroyer of everything, the eternal Father and Mother of the universe, but One who is eternally separate from us and from all souls; and liberation consists in coming near to Him and living in Him. Then there is the other idea of the Impersonal, where all those adjectives are taken away as superfluous, as illogical, and there remains an impersonal, omnipresent Being who cannot be called a knowing being, because knowledge only belongs to the human mind. He cannot be called a thinking being, because that is a process of the weak only. He cannot be called a reasoning being, because reasoning is a

sign of weakness. He cannot be called a creating being, because none creates except in bondage. What bondage has He? None works except for the fulfilment of desires; what desires has He? None works except it be to supply some wants; what wants has He? In the Vedas it is not the word "He" that is used, but "It", for "He" would make an invidious distinction, as if God were a man. (III. 128-29.)

15. Personal God is as much an entity for Himself as we are for ourselves, and no more. God can also be seen as a form, just as we are seen. As men we must have God; as gods we need none. This is why Sri Ramakrishna constantly saw the Divine Mother ever present with him, more real than any other thing around him; but in Samadhi all went but the Self. Personal God comes nearer and nearer until He melts away and there is no more Personal God and no more "I", all is merged in the Self. (VII. 57-58.)

16. A man who understands and believes in the Impersonal—John Stuart Mill, for example —may say that a Personal God is impossible, and cannot be proved. I admit with him that a Personal God cannot be demonstrated. But He is the highest reading of the Impersonal that can be reached by the human intellect, and what else is the universe but various readings of the Absolute? It is like a book before us, and each one

has brought his intellect to read it, and each one has to read it for himself. (II. 337.)

17. All is Brahman, the One without a second; only the Brahman, as unity or absolute, is too much of an abstraction to be loved and worshipped; so the Bhakta chooses the relative aspect of Brahman, that is, Ishwara, the Supreme Ruler. (III. 37.)

18. The Personal God is the same Absolute looked at through the haze of Maya. When we approach Him with the five senses, we can see Him only as the Personal God. The idea is that the Self cannot be objectified. How can the Knower know Itself? But It can cast a shadow, as it were, if that can be called objectification. So the highest form of that shadow, that attempt at objectifying Itself is the Personal God. (V. 266.)

19. The Self is the eternal subject, and we are struggling all the time to objectify that Self. And out of that struggle has come this phenomenal universe and what we call matter, and so on. But these are very weak attempts, and the highest objectification of the Self possible to us is the Personal God. This objectification is an attempt to reveal our own nature. (V. 266.)

20. Man is an infinite circle whose circumference is nowhere, but the centre is located on one spot; and God is an infinite circle whose

circumference is nowhere, but whose centre is everywhere. (II. 33.)

21. Today God is being abandoned by the world because He does not seem to be doing enough for the world. So they say, "Of what good is He?" Shall we look upon God as a mere municipal authority? (VII. 18.)

22. All these forms and ceremonies, these prayers and pilgrimages, these books, bells, candles and priests, are the preparations; they take off the impurities of the soul; and when the soul becomes pure, it naturally wants to get to the mine of purity, God Himself. (II. 46.)

23. We have always heard that every religion insists on our having faith. We have been taught to believe blindly. Well, this idea of blind faith is objectionable, no doubt, but analysing it, we find that behind it is a very great truth.... The mind is not to be ruffled by vain arguments, because arguments will not help us to know God. It is a question of fact, and not of argument. (II. 162.)

24. I have been asked many times, "Why do you use that word, God?" Because it is the best word for our purpose; you cannot find a better word than that, because all the hopes, aspirations and happiness of humanity have been centred in that word. It is impossible now to change the word. Words like these were first coined by

great saints, who realised their import and understood their meaning. But as they become current in society, ignorant people take these words, and the result is that they lose their spirit and glory. The word God has been used from time immemorial, and the idea of this cosmic intelligence, and all that is great and holy is associated with it. (II. 210.)

25. This competition, cruelty, horror and sighs rending hearts day and night, is the state of things in this world of ours. If this be the creation of a God, that God is worse than cruel, worse than any devil that man ever imagined. Aye, says the Vedanta, it is not the fault of God that this partiality exists, that this competition exists. Who makes it? We ourselves. There is a cloud shedding its rain on all fields alike. But it is only the field that is well cultivated, which gets the advantages of the shower; another field, which has not been tilled or taken care of, cannot get that advantage. It is not the fault of the cloud. The mercy of God is eternal and unchangeable; it is we that make the differentiation. But how can this difference of some being born happy and some unhappy be explained? They do nothing to make that difference! Not in this life, but they did in their last birth and the difference is explained by this action in the previous life. (III. 124.)

26. The highest ideal of every man is called God. Ignorant or wise, saint or sinner, man or woman, educated or uneducated, cultivated or uncultivated, to every human being the highest ideals of beauty, of sublimity, and of power, gives us the completest conception of the loving and lovable God. These ideals exist, in some shape or other, in every mind naturally; they form a part and parcel of all our minds. All the active manifestations of human nature are struggles of those ideals to become realised in practical life. (III. 89-90.)

27. Three great gifts we have: first, a human body. (The human mind is the nearest reflection of God, we are "His own image".) Second, the desire to be free. Third, the help of a noble soul who has crossed the ocean of delusion, as a teacher. When you have these three, bless the Lord; you are sure to be free. (VII. 77.)

28. The Lord alone is true; everything else is untrue; everything else should be rejected for the sake of the Lord. Vanity of vanities, all is vanity. Serve the Lord and Him alone. (IV. 60.)

29. Be strong and stand up and seek the God of Love. This is the highest strength. What power is higher than the power of purity? Love and purity govern the world. This love of God cannot be reached by the weak; therefore, be not weak,

either physically, mentally, morally, or spiritually. (IV. 60.)

30. The whole universe is a symbol, and God is the essence behind. (I. 72.)

31. The mountains of today were the oceans of yesterday and will be oceans tomorrow. Everything is in a state of flux; the whole universe is a mass of change. But there is One who never changes, and that is God. (I. 412.)

32. God is an infinitised human being. It is bound to be so, for so long as we are human we must have a human God. (VI. 139.)

33. We have to sense God to be convinced that there is a God. We must sense the facts of religion to know that they are facts. Nothing else, and no amount of reasoning, but our own perceptions can make these things real to us, can make my belief firm as a rock. (IV. 167.)

34. Truth has such a face that anyone who sees that face becomes convinced. The sun does not require any torch to show it; the sun is self-effulgent. If truth requires evidence, what will evidence that evidence? (I. 415.)

35. What is the proof of God? Direct perception, Pratyaksha. The proof of this wall is that I perceive it. God has been perceived by all who want to perceive Him. But this perception is no sense-perception at all; it is supersensuous, superconscious. (I. 415.)

36. This cosmic intelligence is what people call Lord, or God, or Christ, or Buddha, or Brahman, what the materialists perceive as force, and the agnostics as the infinite inexpressible beyond; and we are all parts of that. (II. 231.)

XVII

GURU OR THE SPIRITUAL GUIDE

1. The soul can only receive impulses from another soul, and from nothing else. We may study books all our lives, we may become very intellectual, but in the end, we find that we have not developed at all spiritually. It is not true that a high order of intellectual development always goes hand in hand with a proportionate development of the spiritual side in man.... This inadequacy of books to quicken spiritual growth is the reason why, although almost every one of us can *speak* most wonderfully on spiritual matters, when it comes to action and the living of a spiritual life, we find ourselves awfully deficient. To quicken the spirit, the impulse *must* come from another soul. The person from whose soul such impulse comes is called the Guru—the teacher; and the person to whose soul the impulse is conveyed is called the Shishya—the student.... "The true preacher of religion has to be of wonderful capabilities, and clever shall his hearer be"; and when both of these are really wonderful and extraordinary, then will a splendid spiritual awakening result, and not otherwise. (III. 45-46.)

2. Such is the Guru—"Who has himself

crossed the terrible ocean of life, and without any idea of gain to himself, helps others also to cross the ocean." This is the Guru, and mark that none else can be a Guru. (III. 346.)

3. It is a mysterious law of nature, that as soon as the field is ready, the seed *must* come, as soon as the soul *wants* religion, the transmitter of religious force *must* come. "The seeking sinner meeteth the seeking saviour." When the power that attracts in the receiving soul is full and ripe, the power which answers to the attraction must come. (IV. 22-23.)

4. The real Guru is the one through whom we have our spiritual descent. He is the channel through which the spiritual current flows to us, the link which joins us to the spiritual world. Too much faith in personality has a tendency to produce weakness and idolatry, but intense love for the Guru makes rapid growth possible, he connects us with the internal Guru. Adore your Guru if there be real truth in him; that Guru-bhakti (devotion to the teacher) will quickly lead you to the highest. (VII. 84-85.)

5. If the Brahman is manifested in one man, thousands of men advance, finding their way out in that light. Only the knowers of Brahman are the spiritual teachers of mankind. This is corroborated by all Scriptures and reason too. It is only the selfish Brahmins who have intro-

duced into this country the system of hereditary Gurus, which is against the Vedas and against the Shastras. Hence it is that even through their spiritual practice men do not succeed in perfecting themselves or in realising Brahman. (VI. 464-65.)

6. There are still greater dangers in regard to the *transmitter*, the Guru. There are many who, though immersed in ignorance, yet, in the pride of their hearts, fancy they know everything, and not only do not stop there, but offer to take others on their shoulders; and thus the blind leading the blind, both fall into the ditch. ...The world is full of these. Every one wants to be a teacher, every beggar wants to make a gift of a million dollars! Just as these beggars are ridiculous, so are these teachers. (III. 47.)

7. There is nothing higher and holier than the knowledge which comes to the soul transmitted by a spiritual teacher. If a man has become a perfect Yogi it comes by itself, but it cannot be got in books. You may go and knock your head against the four corners of the world, seek in the Himalayas, the Alps, the Caucasus, the Desert of Gobi or Sahara, or the bottom of the sea, but it will not come, until you find a teacher. (IV. 28.)

8. Get the mercy of God and of His greatest children; these are the two chief ways to God.

The company of these children of light is very hard to get; five minutes in their company will change a whole life, and if you really want it enough, one will come to you, The presence of those who love God makes a place holy, "such is the glory of the children of the Lord". They are He; and when they speak, their words are Scriptures. The place where they have been, becomes filled with their vibrations, and those going there feel them and have a tendency to become holy also. (VII. 10.)

XVIII

HAPPINESS

1. Man thinks foolishly that he can make himself happy, and after years of struggle finds out at last that true happiness consists in killing selfishness and that no one can make him happy except himself. (I. 84.)

2. Nobody is really happy here. If a man be wealthy and have plenty to eat, his digestion is out of order, and he cannot eat. If a man's digestion be good, and he have the digestion of a cormorant, he has nothing to put into his mouth. If he be rich, he has no children. If he be hungry and poor, he has a whole regiment of children, and does not know what to do with them. Why is it so? Because happiness and misery are the obverse and reverse of the same coin; he who takes happiness, must take misery also. We all have this foolish idea that we can have happiness without misery, and it has taken such possession of us that we have no control over the senses. (I. 409.)

3. In some oil mills in India, bullocks are used that go round and round to grind the oil-seed. There is a yoke on the bullock's neck. They have a piece of wood protruding from the yoke, and on that is fastened a wisp of straw.

The bullock is blindfolded in such a way that it can only look forward, and so it stretches its neck to get at the straw; and in doing so, it pushes the piece of wood out a little further; and it makes another attempt with the same result, and yet another, and so on. It never catches the straw, but goes round and round in the hope of getting it, and in so doing grinds out the oil. In the same way you and I who are born slaves of nature, money and wealth, wives and children, are always chasing a wisp of straw, a mere chimera, and going through an innumerable round of lives without obtaining what we seek. The great dream is love, we are all going to love and be loved, we are all going to be happy and never meet with misery, but the more we go towards happiness, the more it goes away from us. (I. 408.)

4. We have seen how happiness is either in the body or in the mind, or in the Atman. With animals, and in the lowest of human beings, who are very much like animals, happiness is all in the body. No man can eat with the same pleasure as a famished dog, or a wolf; so, in the dog and the wolf the happiness is entirely in the body. In men we find a higher plane of happiness, that of thought, and in the Jnani there is the highest plane of happiness in the Self, the Atman. So to the philosopher this knowledge of the Self is

HAPPINESS

of the highest utility, because it gives him the highest happiness possible. Sense gratification or physical things cannot be of the highest utility to him, because he does not find in them the same pleasure that he finds in knowledge itself; and after all, knowledge is the one goal, and is really the highest happiness we know. (III. 19-20.)

5. "Dependence is misery. Independence is happiness." The Advaita is the only system which gives unto man complete possession of himself, takes off all dependence and its associated superstitions, thus making us brave to suffer, brave to do, and in the long run attain to Absolute Freedom. (V. 436.)

6. Can any permanent happiness be given to the world? In the ocean we cannot raise a wave without causing a hollow somewhere else. The sum total of the good things in the world has been the same throughout in its relation to man's need and greed. It cannot be increased or decreased. Take the history of the human race as we know today. Do we not find the same miseries and the same happiness, the same pleasures and pains, the same differences in position? Are not some rich, some poor, some high, some low, some healthy, some unhealthy? All this was the same with the Egyptians, the Greeks and the Romans in ancient times as it is with the

Americans today. So far as the history is known, it has always been the same. (I. 111-12.)

7. We cannot add happiness to this world; similarly, we cannot add pain to it either. The sum total of the energies of pleasure and pain displayed here on earth will be the same throughout. We just push it from this side to the other side, and from that side to this, but it will remain the same, because to remain so is its very nature. This ebb and flow, this rising and falling, is in the world's very nature; it would be as logical to hold otherwise as to say that we may have life without death. (I. 112.)

8. Philosophy insists that there is a joy which is absolute, which never changes. That joy cannot be the joys and pleasures we have in this life, and yet Vedanta shows that everything that is joyful in this life is but a particle of that real joy, because that is the only joy there is. Every moment we are enjoying the absolute bliss, though covered up, misunderstood and caricatured. Wherever there is any blessing, blissfulness, or joy, even the joy of the thief in stealing, it is that Absolute Bliss coming out, only it has become obscured, muddled up, as it were, with all sorts of extraneous conditions, and misunderstood. (II. 166-67.)

9. After every happiness comes misery; they may be far apart or near. The more advanced

the soul, the more quickly does one follow the other. *What we want is neither happiness nor misery.* Both make us forget our true nature; both are chains, one iron, one gold; behind both is the Atman, who knows neither happiness nor misery. (VII. 11.)

10. Happiness presents itself before man, wearing the crown of sorrow on its head. He who welcomes it must also welcome sorrow. (V. 419.)

11. Then alone can death cease when I am one with life, then alone can misery cease when I am one with happiness itself, then alone can error cease when I am one with knowledge itself. (I. 14.)

12. The miseries of the world cannot be cured by physical help only. Until man's nature changes, these physical needs will arise, and miseries will always be felt, and no amount of physical help will cure them completely. The only solution of this problem is to make mankind pure. Ignorance is the mother of all the evil and all the misery we see. Let men have light, let them be pure and spiritually strong and educated, then alone will misery cease in the world, not before. (I. 53.)

13. So long as there is desire no real happiness can come. It is only the contemplative,

witnesslike study of objects that brings to us real enjoyment and happiness. (I. 186.)

14. The animal has its happiness in the senses, the man in his intellect, and the god in spiritual contemplation. It is only to the soul that has attained to this contemplative state that the world really becomes beautiful. To him who desires nothing, and does not mix himself up with them, the manifold changes of nature are one panorama of beauty and sublimity. (I. 186-87.)

XIX

HINDUISM

1. Hinduism indicates one duty, only one, for the human soul. It is to seek to realise the permanent amidst the evanescent. No one presumes to point out any one way in which this may be done. Marriage or non-marriage, good or evil, learning or ignorance, any of these is justified, if it leads to the goal. In this respect lies the great contrast between it and Buddhism, for the latter's outstanding direction is to realise the impermanence of the external, which, broadly speaking, can only be done in one way. Do you recall the story of the young Yogi in the Mahabharata, who prided himself on his psychic powers by burning the bodies of a crow and a crane by his intense will, produced by anger? Do you remember that the young saint went into the town and found first a wife nursing her sick husband and then the butcher Dharmavyadha, both of whom had obtained enlightenment in the path of common faithfulness and duty? (V. 232.)

2. From the high spiritual flights of the Vedanta philosophy, of which the latest discoveries of science seem like echoes, to the low ideas of idolatry with its multifarious mythology, the agnosticism of the Buddhists and the atheism

of the Jains, each and all have a place in the Hindus religion. (I. 6.)

3. To the Hindu, then, the whole world of religions is only a travelling, a coming up of different men and women, through various conditions and circumstances to the same goal. Every religion is only evolving a God out of the material man, and the same God is the inspirer of all of them. Why, then, are there so many contradictions? They are only apparent, says the Hindu. The contradictions come from the same truth adapting itself to the varying circumstances of different natures. (I. 18.)

4. To the Hindu, man is not travelling from error to truth, but from truth to truth, from lower to higher truth. To him all the religions, from the lowest fetishism to the highest absolutism, mean so many attempts of the human soul to grasp and realise the Infinite, each determined by the conditions of its birth and association, and each of these marks a stage of progress; and every soul is a young eagle soaring higher and higher, gathering more and more strength till it reaches the Glorious Sun. (I. 17.)

5. Notwithstanding the differences and controversies existing among our various sects, there are in them too, several grounds of unity. First, almost all of them admit the existence of three things—three entities—Ishvara, Atman and the

Jagat. Ishvara is He who is eternally creating, preserving and destroying the whole universe. Excepting the Sankhyas, all others believe in this. Then the doctrine of the Atman, and the reincarnation of the soul; it maintains that innumerable individual souls having taken body after body again and again, go round and round in the wheel of birth and death according to their respective Karmas; this is Samsaravada or ...the doctrine of rebirth. Then there is this Jagat or universe, without beginning and without end. Though some hold these three as different phases of one only, and some others as three distinctly different entities, and others again in various other ways, yet they are all unanimous in believing in these three. (III. 458-59.)

6. You are hearing every day, and sometimes, I am sorry to say, from men who ought to know better, denunciations of our religion, because it is not at all a conquering religion. To my mind that is the argument why our religion is truer than any other religion, because it never conquered, because it never shed blood, because its mouth always shed on all words of blessing, of peace, words of love and sympathy. It is here and here alone that the ideals of toleration were first preached; and it is here and here alone that toleration and sympathy have become practical; it is theoretical in every other country; it is here

and here alone, that the Hindus build mosques for the Mohammedans and churches for the Christians. (III. 273-74.)

7. The cardinal features of the Hindu religion are founded on the meditative and speculative philosophy and on the ethical teachings contained in the various books of the Vedas, which assert that the universe is infinite in space and eternal in duration. It never had a beginning, and it never had an end. Innumerable have been the manifestations of the power of the Spirit in the realm of matter, of the force of the Infinite in the dominion of the finite, but the Infinite Spirit Itself is self-existent, eternal and unchangeable. The passage of time makes no mark whatever on the dial of eternity. In the supersensuous region which cannot be comprehended at all by the human understanding, there is no past, and there is no future. The Vedas teach that the soul of man is immortal. The body is subject to the law of growth and decay; what grows, must of necessity decay. But the indwelling Spirit is related to the infinite and eternal life; it never had a beginning and it never will have an end. (IV. 188.)

8. Proselytism is tolerated by Hinduism. Any man, whether he be a Shudra or Chandala, can expound philosophy even to a Brahmin. The truth can be learnt from the lowest individual,

no matter to what caste or creed he belongs. (V. 209.)

9. When the Mohammedans first came, we are said—I think, on the authority of Ferishta, the oldest Mohammedan historian—to have been six hundred millions of Hindus. Now we are about two hundred millions. And then every man going out of the Hindu pale is not only a man less, but an enemy the more.

Again, the vast majority of Hindu perverts to Islam and Christianity are perverts by the sword, or the descendants of those. It would be obviously unfair to subject these to disabilities of any kind. As to the case of born aliens, did you say? Why, born aliens have been converted in the past by crowds, and the process is still going on.

In my own opinion, this statement not only applies to original tribes, to outlying nations, and to almost all our conquerors before the Mohammedan conquest, but also to all those castes who had a special origin in the Puranas. I hold that they have been aliens thus adopted.

Ceremonies of expiation are no doubt suitable in the case of willing converts, returning to their Mother-Church, as it were; but on those who were alienated by conquest—as in Kashmir and Nepal—or on strangers wishing to join us, no penance should be imposed. (V. 233-34.)

10. The Hindu does not want to live upon

words and theories. If there are existences beyond the ordinary sensuous existence, he wants to come face to face with them.... The Hindu religion does not consist in struggles and attempts to believe a certain doctrine or dogma, but in realising—not in believing, but in being and becoming. (I. 13.)

XX

HINDUS

1. In India there never was any religious persecution by the Hindus, but only that wonderful reverence, which they have for all the religions of the world. They sheltered a portion of the Hebrews, when they were driven out of their own country; and the Malabar Jews remain as a result. They received at another time the remnant of the Persians, when they were almost annihilated; and they remain to this day, as a part of us and loved by us, as the modern Parsees of Bombay. There were Christians who claimed to have come with St. Thomas, the disciple of Jesus Christ; they were allowed to settle in India and hold their own opinions; and a colony of them is even now in existence in India. And this spirit of toleration has not died out. It will not and cannot die there. (I. 391.)

2. You may be a dualist, and I may be a monist. You may believe that you are the eternal servant of God, and I may declare that I am one with God Himself; yet both of us are good Hindus. How is that possible? Read then एकं सद्विप्रा बहुधा वदन्ति—"That which exists is One; sages call It by various names". (III. 113.)

3. One peculiarity of the Hindu mind is that

it always inquires for the last possible generalisation, leaving the details to be worked out afterwards. The question is raised in the Vedas, "What is that, knowing which we shall know everything?" Thus, all books, and all philosophies that have been written, have been only to prove *that* by knowing which everything is known. (I. 148-49.)

4. The Hindus were bold, to their credit be it said, bold thinkers in all their ideas, so bold that one spark of their thought frightens the so-called bold thinkers of the West. Well has it been said by Prof. Max Müller about these thinkers, that they climbed up to heights where their lungs only could breathe, and where those of other beings would have burst. These brave people followed reason wherever it led them, no matter at what cost, never caring what society would think about them, or talk about them, but what they thought was right and true, they preached and they talked. (I. 346-47.)

5. The ancient Hindus were wonderful scholars, veritable living encyclopaedias. They said, "Knowledge in books and money in other people's hands is like no knowledge and no money at all". (VII. 40.)

6. With the Hindus you will find one national idea—spirituality. In no other religion, in no other sacred books of the world, will you find so

much energy spent in defining the idea of God. They tried to define the idea of soul so that no earthly touch might mar it. The spiritual must be divine; and spirit understood as spirit must not be made into a man. (II. 372.)

7. The Aryan man was always seeking Divinity inside his own self. It became, in course of time, natural, characteristic. It is remarkable in their art and in their commonest dealings. Even at the present time, if we take a European picture of a man in a religious attitude, the painter always makes his subject point his eyes upwards, looking outside of nature for God, looking up into the skies. In India, on the other hand, the religious attitude is always presented by making the subject close his eyes. He is, as it were, looking inward. (VI. 3-4.)

8. The word Hindu, by which it is the fashion nowadays to style ourselves, has lost all its meaning, for this word merely meant those who lived on the other side of the river Indus (in Sanskrit Sindhu). This name was murdered into Hindu, by the ancient Persians, and all people living on the other side of the river Sindhu were called by them Hindus. Thus this word has come down to us, and during the Mohammedan rule we took up the word ourselves. (III. 118.)

9. You are Hindus, and there is the instinctive belief in you that life is eternal. Sometimes

I have young men come and talk to me about atheism; I do not believe a Hindu can become an atheist. He may read European books, and persuade himself he is a materialist, but it is only for a time. It is not in your blood. You cannot believe what is not in your constitution; it would be a hopeless task for you. Do not attempt that sort of thing. I once attempted it when I was a boy; but it could not be. (III. 304.)

XXI

THE HOUSEHOLDER'S LIFE

1. The householder should be devoted to God; the knowledge of God should be the goal of his life. Yet he must work constantly, perform all his duties; he must give up the fruits of his actions to God. (I. 42.)

2. Do your Svadharma—this is truth, the truth of truths.... Of course, do not do any wrong, do not injure or tyrannise over any one, but try to do good to others as much as you can. But passively to submit to wrong done by others is a sin—with the householder. He must try to pay them back in their own coin then and there. (V. 448.)

3. The householder must earn money with great effort and enthusiasm, and by that must support and bring comforts to his own family and to others, and perform good works as far as possible. If you cannot do that, how do you profess to be a man? You are not a householder even—what to talk of Moksha for you! (V. 448-49.)

4. The rule for a householder about the expenditure of his income is, one-fourth of the income for his family, one-fourth for charity, one-fourth to be saved, one-fourth for self. (VI. 114.)

5. If a man retires from the world to worship God, he must not think that those who live in the world and work for the good of the world are not worshipping God; neither must those who live in the world, for wife and children, think that those who give up the world are low vagabonds. Each is great in his own place. (I. 45.)

6. The West regards marriage as consisting in all that lies beyond the legal tie, while in India it is thought of as a bond thrown by society round two people, to unite them together for all eternity. Those two must wed each other, whether they will or not, in life after life. Each acquires half of all the merit of the other. And if one seems in this life to have fallen hopelessly behind, it is for the other only to wait and beat time, till he or she catches up again. (VIII. 276.)

7. Chastity is the first virtue in man or woman, and the man who, however he may have strayed away, cannot be brought to the right path by a gentle and loving and chaste wife, is indeed very rare. The world is not yet as bad as that. We hear much about brutal husbands all over the world and about the impurity of men, but is it not true that there are quite as many brutal and impure women as men? If all women were as good and pure as their own constant assertions would lead one to believe, I am perfectly satisfied that there would not be one impure man in

the world. What brutality is there which purity and chastity cannot conquer? A good, chaste wife, who thinks of every other man except her own husband as her child and has the attitude of a mother towards all men, will grow so great in the power of her purity that there cannot be a single man, however brutal, who will not breathe an atmosphere of holiness in her presence. Similarly, every husband must look upon all women, except his own wife, in the light of his own mother or daughter or sister. That man, again, who wants to be a teacher of religion must look upon every woman as his mother, and always behave towards her as such. (I. 67-68.)

8. The householder is the centre of life and society. It is a worship for him to acquire and spend wealth nobly, for the householder who struggles to become rich by *good* means and for *good* purposes is doing practically the same thing for the attainment of salvation as the anchorite does in his cell when he is praying, for in them we see only the different aspects of the same virtue of self-surrender and self-sacrifice prompted by the feeling of devotion to God and to all that is His. (I. 46.)

9. Do you ask anything from your children in return for what you have given them? It is your duty to work for them, and there the matter ends. In whatever you do for a particular person, a

city, or a state, assume the same attitude towards it as you have towards your children—expect nothing in return. If you can invariably take the position of a giver, in which everything given by you is a free offering to the world, without any thought of return, then will your work bring you no attachment. (I. 59.)

10. My Master used to say, "Look upon your children as a nurse does". The nurse will take your baby and fondle it and play with it and behave towards it as gently as if it were her own child; but as soon as you give her notice to quit she is ready to start off bag and baggage.... Everything in the shape of attachment is forgotten; it will not cause the ordinary nurse the least pang to leave your children and take up other children. Even so are you to be with all that you consider your own. You are the nurse, and if you believe in God, believe that all these things which you consider yours are really His. (I. 88-89.)

11. To his enemies the householder must be a hero. Them he must resist. That is the duty of the householder. He must not sit down in a corner and weep, and talk nonsense about non-resistance. If he does not show himself a hero to his enemies he has not done his duty. And to his friends and relatives he must be as gentle as a lamb. (I. 44.)

12. The householder must speak the truth, and speak gently, using words which people like, which will do good to others; nor should he talk of the business of other men. (I. 46.)

13. He must struggle to acquire a good name by all means. He must not gamble, he must not move in the company of the wicked, he must not tell lies, and must not be the cause of trouble to others. (I. 46.)

XXII

IDEAL WOMANHOOD

1. The great Aryans, Buddha among the rest, have always put woman in an equal position with man. For them sex in religion did not exist. In the Vedas and Upanishads, women taught the highest truths and received the same veneration as men. (VIII. 28.)

2. Buddha, however, recognised woman's right to an equal place in religion and his first and one of his greatest disciples was his own wife, who became the head of the whole Buddhistic movement among the women of India. (VII. 78.)

3. In the records of the saints in India there is the unique figure of the prophetess. In the Christian creed they are all prophets, while in India the holy women occupy a conspicuous place in the holy books. (VIII. 207.)

4. Do you remember how Yajnavalkya was questioned at the court of King Janaka? His principal examiner was Vachaknavi, the maiden orator—Brahmavadini, as the word of the day was. "Like two shining arrows in the hand of the skilled archer," she says, "are my questions." Her sex is not even commented upon. Again, could anything be more complete than the equality of

boys and girls in our old forest universities? Read our Sanskrit dramas—read the story of Shakuntala, and see if Tennyson's "Princess" has anything to teach us! (V. 230.)

5. The Aryan and Semitic ideals of woman have always been diametrically opposed. Amongst the Semites the presence of woman is considered dangerous to devotion, and she may not perform any religious function, even such as the killing of a bird for food: according to the Aryan a man cannot perform a religious action without a wife. (V. 229.)

6. There is no chance for the welfare of the world unless the condition of women is improved. It is not possible for a bird to fly on only one wing.

Hence, in the Ramakrishna Incarnation, the acceptance of a woman as the Guru, hence His practising in the woman's garb and frame of mind, hence too His preaching the Motherhood of women as representations of the Divine Mother. (VI. 328.)

7. If you do not allow one to become a lion, he will become a fox. Women are a power, only now it is more for evil because man oppresses woman; she is the fox, but when she is no longer oppressed, she will become the lion. (VII. 22.)

8. The best thermometer to the progress of a nation is its treatment of its women. In ancient

Greece there was absolutely no difference in the state of man and woman. The idea of perfect equality existed. No Hindu can be a priest until he is married, the idea being that a single man is only half a man, and imperfect. The idea of perfect womanhood is perfect independence. The central ideal of the life of a modern Hindu lady is her chastity. The wife is the centre of a circle, the fixity of which depends upon her chastity. It was the extreme of this idea which caused Hindu widows to be burnt. The Hindu women are very spiritual and very religious, perhaps more so than any other women in the world. If we can preserve these beautiful characteristics and at the same time develop the intellects of our women, the Hindu woman of the future will be the ideal woman of the world. (VIII. 198.)

9. In my opinion, a race must first cultivate a great respect for motherhood, through the sanctification and inviolability of marriage, before it can attain to the ideal of perfect chastity. The Roman Catholics and the Hindus, holding marriage sacred and inviolate, have produced great chaste men and women of immense power. To the Arab, marriage is a contract or a forceful possession, to be dissolved at will, and we do not find there the development of the idea of the virgin or the Brahmacharin. Modern Buddhism

—having fallen among races who had not yet come up to the evolution of marriage—has made a travesty of monasticism. So, until there is developed in Japan a great and sacred ideal about marriage (apart from mutual attraction and love), I do not see how there can be great monks and nuns. As you have come to see that the glory of life is chastity, so my eyes also have been opened to the necessity of this great sanctification for the vast majority, in order that a few lifelong chaste powers may be produced. (V. 180.)

10. At the present time God should be worshipped as "Mother", the Infinite Energy. This will lead to purity, and tremendous energy will come here in America. Here no temples weigh us down, no one suffers as they do in poorer countries. Woman has suffered for aeons, and that has given her infinite patience and infinite perseverance. She holds on to an idea. It is this which makes her the support of even superstitious religions and of the priests in every land, and it is this that will free her. We have to become Vedantists and live this grand thought; the masses must get it, and only in free America can this be done. In India these ideas were brought out by individuals like Buddha, Shankara, and others, but the masses did not retain them. The new cycle must see the masses living

Vedanta, and this will have to come through women.

"Keep the beloved beautiful Mother in the heart of your hearts with all care."

"Throw out everything but the tongue, keep that to say, 'Mother, Mother!'"

"Let no evil counsellors enter; let you and me, my heart, alone see Mother."

"Thou art beyond all that lives!"

"My Moon of life, my Soul of soul!" (VII. 95.)

11. You have not yet understood the wonderful significance of Mother's life—none of you. But gradually you will know. Without Shakti (Power) there is no regeneration for the world. Why is it that our country is the weakest and the most backward of all countries? Because Shakti is held in dishonour there. Mother has been born to revive that wonderful Shakti in India; and making her the nucleus, once more will Gargis and Maitreyis be born in the world. Dear brother, you understand little now. But by degrees you will come to know it all. Hence it is her Math that I want first.... Without the grace of Shakti nothing is to be accomplished. What do I find in America and Europe?—the worship of Shakti, the worship of Power. Yet they worship Her ignorantly through sense-gratification. Imagine, then, what a lot of good they will achieve who will worship Her with all

purity, in a Sattvika spirit, looking upon Her as their mother. I am coming to understand things clearer every day, my insight is opening out more and more. Hence we must first build a Math for Mother. First Mother and her daughters, then Father and his sons—can you understand this? ... To me, Mother's grace is a hundred thousand times more valuable than Father's. Mother's grace, Mother's blessings are all paramount to me.... (VII. 482.)

12. "I know that the race that produced Sita —even if it only dreamt of her—has a reverence for woman that is unmatched on the earth. There is many a burden bound with legal tightness on the shoulders of Western women that is utterly unknown to ours. We have our wrongs and our exceptions certainly, but so have they. We must never forget that all over the globe the general effort is to express love and tenderness and uprightness, and that national customs are only the nearest vehicles of this expression. With regard to the domestic virtues I have no hesitation in saying that our Indian methods have in many ways the advantage over all others."

"Then have our women any problems at all, Swamiji?"

"Of course, they have many and grave problems, but none that are not to be solved by that magic word education. The true education, however, is not yet conceived of amongst us."

"And how would you define that?"

"I never define anything", said the Swami, smiling. "Still, it may be described as a development of faculty, not an accumulation of words, or as a training of individuals to will rightly and efficiently. So shall we bring to the need of India great fearless women—women worthy to continue the traditions of Sanghamitta, Lila, Ahalya Bai, and Mira Bai—women fit to be mothers of heroes, because they are pure and selfless, strong with the strength that comes of touching the feet of God." (V. 231.)

13. I should very much like our women to have your intellectuality, but not if it must be at the cost of purity. I admire you for all that you know, but I dislike the way that you cover what is bad with roses and call it good. Intellectuality is not the highest good. Morality and spirituality are the things for which we strive. Our women are not so learned, but they are more pure.

To all women every man save her husband should be as her son. To all men every women save his own wife should be as his mother. When I look about me and see what you call gallantry my soul is filled with disgust. Not until you learn to ignore the question of sex and to meet on a ground of common humanity will your women really develop. Until then they are playthings, nothing more. All this is the cause of divorce. Your men bow low and offer a chair, but in another breath they offer compliments. They say, Oh, madam, how beautiful are your eyes! What right have they to do this? How dare a man venture so far, and how can your women permit it? Such things develop the less noble side of humanity. They do not tend to nobler ideals.

We should not think that we are men and women, but only that we are human beings, born to cherish and to help one another. No sooner are a young man and a young woman left alone than he pays compliments to her, and perhaps before he takes a wife he has courted two hundred women. Bah! If I belonged to the marrying set I could find a woman to love, without all that!

When I was in India and saw these things from the outside I was told it was all right, it was mere pleasantry, and I believed it. But I have travelled since then, and I know it is not right. It is wrong, only you of the West shut your eyes and call it good. The trouble with the nations of the West is that they are young, foolish, fickle and wealthy. What mischief can come of one of these qualities, but when all these three, all four, are combined, beware! (V. 412-13.)

14. Then, religion comes into the question; the Hindu religion comes in as a comfort. For, mind you, our religion teaches that marriage is something bad, it is only for the weak. The very spiritual man or woman would not marry at all. So the religious woman says, "Well, the Lord has given me a better chance. What is the use of marrying? Thank God, worship God, what is the use of my loving man?" (VIII. 65-66.)

15. Next is the worship of woman (in America). This worship of Shakti is not lust, but is that Shakti-Puja, that worship of the Kumari (virgin) and the Sadhava (the married woman whose husband is living), which is done in Varanasi, Kalighat and other holy places. It is the worship of the Shakti, not in mere thought, not in imagination, but in actual, visible form. Our Shakti-worship is only in the holy places, and at certain times only is it performed; but theirs is in every place and always, for days, weeks, months and years. Foremost is the woman's state, foremost is her dress, her seat, her food, her wants and her comforts; the first honours in all respects are accorded to her. Not to speak of the nobleborn, not to speak of the young and the fair, it is the worship of any and every woman, be she an acquaintance or a stranger. (V. 506.)

16. Just as centres have to be started for men,

so also centres have to be started for teaching women. Brahmacharinis of education and character should take up the task of teaching at these different centres. History and the Puranas, house-keeping and the arts, the duties of home-life and principles that make for the development of an ideal character, have to be taught with the help of modern science, and the female students must be trained up in ethical and spiritual life. We must see to their growing up as ideal matrons of home in time. The children of such mothers will make further progress in the virtues that distinguish the mothers. It is only in the homes of educated and pious mothers that great men are born. And you have reduced your women to something like manufacturing machines; alas, for heaven's sake, is this the outcome of your education? The uplift of the women, the awakening of the masses, must come first, and then only can any real good come about for the country, for India. (VI. 489-90.)

17. Wife—the co-religionist. Hundreds of ceremonies the Hindu has to perform, and not one can be performed if he has not a wife. You see the priests tie them up together, and they go round temples and make very great pilgrimages together.

Rama gave up his body and joined Sita in the other world.

Sita—the pure, the pure, the all-suffering!

Sita is the name in India for everything that is good, pure, and holy; everything that in woman we call woman.

Sita—the patient, all-suffering, ever-faithful, ever-pure wife! Through all the suffering she had, there was not one harsh word against Rama.

Sita never returned injury.

Be Sita! (VI. 102-03.)

18. In the West women rule; all influence and power are theirs. If bold and talented women like yourself, versed in Vedanta, go to England to preach, I am sure that every year hundreds of men and women will become blessed by adopting the religion of the land of Bharata. If any one like you go, England will be stirred, what to speak of America! If an Indian woman in Indian dress preach the religion which fell from the lips of the Rishis of India—I see a prophetic vision—there will rise a great wave which will inundate the whole Western world. Will there be no woman in the land of Maitreyi, Khana, Lilavati, Savitri, and Ubhayabharati, who will venture to do this? (VI. 485-86.)

19. Liberty is the first condition of growth. It is wrong, a thousand times wrong, if any of you dares to say, "I will work out the salvation of this woman or child". I am asked again and again, what I think of the widow problem and

IDEAL WOMANHOOD

what I think of the woman question. Let me answer once for all—am I a widow that you ask me that nonsense? Am I a woman that you ask me that question again and again? Who are you to solve women's problems? Are you the Lord God that you should rule over every widow and every woman? Hands off! They will solve their own problems. (III. 246.)

20. Women must be put in a position to solve their own problems in their own way. No one can or ought to do this for them. And our Indian women are as capable of doing it as any in the world. (V. 229-30.)

21. Disciple: But, sir, how would you get now in this country learned and virtuous women like Gargi, Khana or Lilavati?

Swamiji: Do you think women of the type don't exist now in the country? Still on this sacred soil of India, this land of Sita and Savitri, among women may be found such character, such spirit of service, such affection, compassion, contentment and reverence, as I could not find anywhere else in the world! In the West, the women did not very often seem to me to be women at all, they appeared to be quite the replicas of men! Driving vehicles, drudging in offices, attending schools, doing professional duties! In India alone the sight of feminine modesty and reserve soothes the eye! With such materials of great promise, you could not, alas, work out their uplift! You did not try to infuse the light of knowledge into them! For if they get the right sort of education, they may well turn out to be the ideal women in the world. (VI. 491.)

22. With such an education women will solve their own problems. They have all the time been trained in helplessness, servile dependence on others, and so they are good only to weep their eyes out at the slightest approach of a mishap or danger. Along with other things they should acquire the spirit of valour and heroism. In the present day it has become necessary for them also to learn self-defence. See how grand was the Queen of Jhansi! (V. 342.)

23. Well, I am almost at my wit's end to see the women of this country (U.S.A.). They take me to the shops and everywhere, as if I were a child. They do all sorts of work—I cannot do even a sixteenth part of what they do. They are like Lakshmi (the Goddess of Fortune) in beauty, and like Saraswati (the Goddess of Learning) in virtues—they are the Divine Mother incarnate, and worshipping them, one verily attains perfection in everything. Great God! Are we to be counted among men? If I can raise a thousand such Madonnas—Incarnations of the Divine Mother—in our country, before I die, I shall

die in peace. Then only will your countrymen become worthy of their name....

I am really struck with wonder to see the women here. How gracious the Divine Mother is on them! Most wonderful women, these! They are about to corner the men who have been nearly worsted in the competition. It is all through Thy grace, O Mother!...I shall not rest till I root out this distinction of sex. Is there any sex-distinction in the Atman? Out with the differentiation between men and women—all is Atman! Give up the identification with the body, and stand up! Say, अस्ति, अस्ति "Everything is!" —cherish positive thoughts. (VI. 272-73.)

XXIII

IMAGE WORSHIP

1. God is eternal, without any form, omnipresent. To think of Him as possessing any form is blasphemy. But the secret of image worship is that you are trying to develop your vision of Divinity in one thing. (VII. 411.)

2. Of the principal religions of the world we see Vedantism, Buddhism and certain forms of Christianity freely using images; only two religions, Mohammedanism and Protestantism, refuse such help. Yet the Mohammedans use the graves of their saints and martyrs almost in the place of images; and the Protestants, in rejecting all concrete helps to religion, are drifting away every year farther and farther from spirituality. (III. 61.)

3. All of you have been taught to believe in an omnipresent God. Try to think of it. How few of you can have any idea of what omnipresence means! If you struggle hard, you will get something like the idea of ocean, or of the sky, or of a vast stretch of green earth, or of a desert. All these are material images, and so long as you cannot conceive of the abstract *as* abstract, of the ideal *as* the ideal, you will have to resort to these forms, these material images.

It does not make much difference whether these images are inside or outside the mind. We are all born idolaters, and idolatry is good, because it is in the nature of man. Who can get beyond it? Only the perfect man, the God-man. The rest are all idolaters. So long as we see the universe before us, with its forms and shapes, we are all idolaters. This is a gigantic symbol we are worshipping. He who says that he is the body, is a born idolater. We are spirit, spirit that has no form or shape, spirit that is infinite, and not matter. Therefore any one who cannot grasp the abstract, who cannot think of himself as he is, except in and through matter, as the body, is an idolater. And yet how people fight among themselves, calling one another idolaters! In other words, each says, his idol is right, and the others' are wrong. (II. 40.)

4. Two sorts of persons never require any image—the human animal who never thinks of any religion, and the perfected being who has passed through these stages. Between these two points all of us require some sort of ideal, outside and inside. (IV. 45.)

5. It is very easy to say "Don't be personal", but the same man who says so is generally most personal. His attachment for particular men and women is very strong; it does not leave him when they die, he wants to follow them beyond

death. That is idolatry; it is the seed, the very cause of idolatry, and the cause being there it will come out in some form. Is it not better to have a personal attachment to an image of Christ or Buddha than to an ordinary man or woman? (IV. 46.)

6. It has been a trite saying, that idolatry is wrong, and every man swallows it at the present time without questioning. I once thought so, and to pay the penalty of that I had to learn my lesson sitting at the feet of a man who realised everything through idols; I allude to Ramakrishna Paramahamsa. Take a thousand idols more if you can produce Ramakrishna Paramahamsas through idol worship, and may God speed you! (III. 218.)

7. The Christian thinks that when God came in the form of a dove it was all right, but if He comes in the form of a fish, as the Hindus say, it is very wrong and superstitious. The Jews think if an idol be made in the form of a chest with two angels sitting on it, and a book on it, it is all right, but if it is in the form of a man or a woman, it is awful. The Mohammedans think that when they pray, if they try to form a mental image of the temple with the Caaba, the black stone in it, and turn towards the west, it is all right, but if you form the image in the

IMAGE WORSHIP

shape of a church it is idolatry. This is the defect of image worship. (IV. 44-45.)

8. We may worship anything by seeing God *in* it, if we can forget the idol and see God there. We must not project any image upon God. But we may fill any image with that Life which is God. Only forget the image, and you are right enough—for "out of Him comes everything". He is everything. We may worship a picture as God, but not God as the picture. God in the picture is right, but the picture as God is wrong. God *in* the image is perfectly right. There is no danger there. This is the real worship of God. (IV. 47.)

9. "External worship, material worship," say the scriptures, "is the lowest stage; struggling to rise high, mental worship is the next stage, but the highest stage is when the Lord has been realised." Mark, the same earnest man who is kneeling before the idol tells you: "Him the sun cannot express, nor the moon, nor the stars, the lightning cannot express Him, nor what we speak of as fire; through Him they shine." But he does not abuse any one's idol or call its worship sin. He recognises in it a necessary stage of life. "The Child is Father of the man." Would it be right for an old man to say that childhood is a sin or youth a sin? (I. 16-17.)

10. Unity in variety is the plan of nature, and

the Hindu has recognised it. Every other religion lays down certain fixed dogmas, and tries to force society to adopt them. It places before society only one coat which must fit Jack and John and Henry, all alike. If it does not fit John or Henry, he must go without a coat to cover his body. The Hindus have discovered that the absolute can only be realised, or thought of, or stated, through the relative, and the images, crosses and crescents are simply so many symbols—so many pegs to hang the spiritual ideas on. It is not that this help is necessary for every one, but those that do not need it have no right to say that it is wrong. Nor is it compulsory in Hinduism. (I. 17.)

11. Idolatry in India does not mean anything horrible. It is not the mother of harlots. On the other hand, it is the attempt of undeveloped minds to grasp high spiritual truths. The Hindus have their faults, they sometimes have their exceptions; but mark this, they are always for punishing their own bodies, and never for cutting the throats of their neighbours. If the Hindu fanatic burns himself on the pyre, he never lights the fire of Inquisition. And even this cannot be laid at the door of his religion any more than the burning of witches can be laid at the door of Christianity. (I. 17-18.)

12. Superstition is a great enemy of man, but bigotry is worse. Why does a Christian go to

church? Why is the cross holy? Why is the face turned toward the sky in prayer? Why are there so many images in the Catholic Church? Why are there so many images in the minds of Protestants when they pray? My brethren, we can no more think about anything without a mental image than we can live without breathing. By the law of association the material image calls up the mental idea and vice versa. This is why the Hindu uses an external symbol when he worships. He will tell you, it helps to keep his mind fixed on the Being to whom he prays. He knows as well as you do that the image is not God, is not omnipresent. After all, how much does omnipresence mean to almost the whole world? It stands merely as a word, a symbol. Has God superficial area? If not, when we repeat that word "omnipresent", we think of the extended sky or of space, that is all. (I. 15-16.)

13. Man is to become divine by realising the divine. Idols, or temples or churches or books are only the supports, the helps, of his spiritual childhood; but on and on he must progress. (I. 16.)

14. Therefore, we should get rid of these childish notions. We should get beyond the prattle of men who think that religion is merely a mass of frothy words, that it is only a system of doctrines; to whom religion is only a little

intellectual assent or dissent; to whom religion is believing in certain words which their own priests tell them; to whom religion is something which their forefathers believed; to whom religion is a certain form of ideas and superstitions to which they cling, because they are their national superstitions. We should get beyond all these, and look at humanity as one vast organism, slowly coming towards light—a wonderful plant, slowly unfolding itself to that wonderful truth which is called God—and the first gyrations, the first motions, towards this are always through matter and through ritual. (II. 40-41.)

XXIV

INCARNATION

1. Higher and nobler than all ordinary ones, are another set of teachers, the Avataras of Ishvara, in the world. They can transmit spirituality with a touch, even with a mere wish. The lowest and the most degraded characters become in one second saints at their command. They are the Teachers of all teachers, the highest manifestations of God through man. We cannot see God except through them. We cannot help worshipping them, and indeed they are the only ones whom we are bound to worship. (III. 53.)

2. God understands human failings and becomes man to do good to humanity. "Whenever virtue subsides and wickedness prevails I manifest Myself. To establish virtue, to destroy evil, to save the good I come from Yuga to Yuga." "Fools deride Me who have assumed the human form, without knowing My real nature as the Lord of the universe." Such is Sri Krishna's declaration in the Gita on Incarnation. "When a huge tidal wave comes," says Sri Ramakrishna, "all the little brooks and ditches become full to the brim without any effort or consciousness on their own part; so when an Incarnation comes, a tidal wave of spirituality

breaks upon the world, and people feel spirituality almost full in the air." (III. 55-56.)

3. What are we but floating wavelets in the eternal current of events, irresistibly moved forward and onward and incapable of rest? But you and I are only little things, bubbles. There are always some giant waves in the ocean of affairs; and in you and me the life of the past race has been embodied only a little; but there are giants who embody, as it were, almost the whole of the past and who stretch out their hands for the future. These are the signposts here and there, which point to the march of humanity; these are verily gigantic, their shadows covering the earth —they stand undying, eternal! (IV. 139.)

4. As it has been said... "No man hath seen God at any time, but through the Son." And that is true. And where shall we see God but in the Son? It is true that you and I, and the poorest of us, the meanest even, embody that God, even reflect that God. The vibration of light is everywhere, omnipresent, but we have to strike the light of the lamp before we can see the light. The omnipresent God of the universe cannot be seen until He is reflected by these giant lamps of the earth—the Prophets, the Man-Gods, the Incarnations, the embodiments of God. (III. 139.)

5. Personal God is necessary and at the same time we know that instead of and better than

vain imaginations of a Personal God, ... we have in this world, living and walking in our midst, living Gods, now and then. These are more worthy of worship than any imaginary God, any creation of our imagination, that is to say, any idea of God which we can form. Sri Krishna is much greater than any idea of God you or I can have. Buddha is a much higher idea, a more living and idolised idea, than the ideal you or I can conceive of in our minds, and therefore it is that they always command the worship of mankind, even to the exclusion of all imaginary deities. This our sages knew, and therefore left it open to all Indian people to worship such great personages, such Incarnations. (III. 251.)

6. "Wherever an extraordinary spiritual power is manifested by external man, know that I am there; it is from Me that that manifestation comes." That leaves the door open for the Hindu to worship the Incarnations of all the countries in the world. The Hindu can worship any sage and any saint from any country whatsoever, and as a fact we know that we go and worship many times in the churches of the Christians, and many, many times in the Mohammedan mosques, and that is good. (III. 251.)

7. Therefore, it is absolutely necessary to worship God as man, and blessed are those races which have such a "God-man" to worship.

Christians have such a God-Man in Christ. That is the natural way to see God; see God in man. All our ideas of God are concentrated there. (IV. 31.)

8. We talk of principles, we think of theories, and that is all right; but every thought and every movement, every one of our actions, shows that we can understand the principle when it comes to us through a person. We can grasp an idea only when it comes to us through a materialised ideal person. We can understand the precept only through the example. Would to God that all of us were so developed that we would not require any example, would not require any person. But that we are not; and, naturally, the vast majority of mankind have put their souls at the feet of these extraordinary personalities, the Prophets, the Incarnations of God—Incarnations worshipped by the Christians, by the Buddhists, and by the Hindus. (IV. 121.)

9. The Absolute cannot be worshipped, so we must worship a manifestation, such a one as has our nature. Jesus had our nature; he became the Christ; so can we and so *must* we. Christ and Buddha were the names of a state to be attained; Jesus and Gautama were the persons to manifest it. (VII. 29.)

10. Our salutations go to all the past Prophets, whose teachings and lives we have inherited,

INCARNATION

whatever might have been their race, clime or creed! Our salutations go to all those Godlike men and women, who are working to help humanity, whatever be their birth, colour or race! Our salutations to those who are coming in the future—living Gods—to work unselfishly for our descendants! (IV. 153.)

XXV

INDIA—CAUSE OF HER DEGENERATION

1. In our sight, here in India, there are several dangers. Of these, the two, Scylla and Charybdis, rank materialism and its opposite, arrant superstition, must be avoided. There is the man today who after drinking the cup of Western wisdom, thinks that he knows everything. He laughs at the ancient sages. All Hindu thought to him is arrant trash, philosophy, mere child's prattle, and religion, the superstition of fools. On the other hand, there is the man educated, but a sort of monomaniac, who runs to the other extreme, and wants to explain the omen of this and that. He has philosophical and metaphysical, and Lord knows what other puerile explanations for every superstition that belongs to his peculiar race, or his peculiar gods, or his peculiar village. Every little village superstition is to him a mandate of the Vedas, and upon the carrying out of it, according to him, depends the national life. You must beware of this. (III. 278.)

2. First bread and then religion. We stuff them too much with religion, when the poor fellows have been starving. No dogmas will satisfy the cravings of hunger. There are two curses here, first our weakness, secondly, our hatred, our

dried-up hearts. You may talk doctrines by the millions, you may have sects by the hundreds of millions; aye, but it is nothing until you have the heart to feel; feel for them as your Veda teaches you, till you find they are parts of your bodies, till you realise that you and they, the poor and the rich, the saint and the sinner, are all parts of One Infinite Whole, which you call Brahman. (III. 432.)

3. I consider that the great national sin is the neglect of the masses, and that is one of the causes of our downfall. No amount of politics would be of any avail until the masses in India are once more well educated, well fed, and well cared for. (V. 222-23.)

4. If you grind down the people, you will suffer. We in India are suffering the vengeance of God. Look upon these things. They ground down those poor people for their own wealth, they heard not the voice of distress, they ate from gold and silver when the people cried for bread, and the Mohammedans came upon them slaughtering and killing: slaughtering and killing they overran them. India has been conquered again and again for years, and last and worst of all came the Englishman. You look about India, what has the Hindu left? Wonderful temples, everywhere. What has the Mohammedan left? Beautiful palaces. What has

the Englishman left? Nothing but mounds of broken brandy bottles! And God has had no mercy upon my people because they had no mercy. By their cruelty they degraded the populace; and when they needed them, the common people had no strength to give for their aid. If man cannot believe in the Vengeance of God, he certainly cannot deny the Vengeance of History. (VII. 279-80.)

5. We speak of many things, parrotlike, but never do them; speaking and not doing has become a habit with us. What is the cause of this? Physical weakness. This sort of weak brain is not able to do anything; we must strengthen it. (III. 242.)

6. Our nation is totally lacking in the faculty of organisation. It is this one drawback which produces all sorts of evil. We are altogether averse to making a common cause for anything. The first requisite for organisation is obedience. (VI. 322-23.)

7. We would do nothing ourselves and would scoff at others who try to do something—this is the bane that has brought about our downfall as a nation. Want of sympathy and lack of energy are at the root of all misery, and you must therefore give these two up. Who but the Lord knows what potentialities there are in

particular individuals—let all have opportunities, and leave the rest to the Lord. (VI. 359.)

8. Nowadays everybody blames those who constantly look back to the past. It is said that so much looking back to the past is the cause of all India's woes. To me, on the contrary, it seems that the opposite is true. So long as they forgot the past, the Hindu nation remained in a state of stupor; and as soon as they have begun to look into the past, there is on every side a fresh manifestation of life. It is out of this past that the future has to be moulded, this past will become the future. (IV. 324.)

9. The more the Hindus study the past, the more glorious will be their future, and whoever tries to bring the past to the door of every one, is a great benefactor to his nation. The degeneration of India came not because the laws and customs of the ancient were bad, but because they were not allowed to be carried to their legitimate conclusions. (IV. 324.)

10. Whether we are in the state of Sattvika calmness, beyond all pleasure and pain, and past all work and activity, or whether we are in the lowest Tamasika state, lifeless, passive, dull as dead matter, and doing no work, because there is no power in us to do it, and are, thus, silently and by degrees, getting rotten and corrupted within—I seriously ask you this question and

demand an answer. Ask your mind, and you shall know what the reality is. (V. 451.)

11. No man, no nation, my son, can hate others and live. India's doom was sealed the very day they invented the word MLECHCHHA and stopped from communion with others. Take care how you foster that idea. It is good to talk glibly about the Vedanta, but how hard to carry out even its least precepts! (V. 52.)

12. No religion on earth preaches the dignity of humanity in such a lofty strain as Hinduism, and no religion on earth treads upon the necks of the poor and the low in such a fashion as Hinduism. The Lord has shown me that religion is not in fault, but it is the Pharisees and Sadducees in Hinduism, hypocrites, who invent all sorts of engines of tyranny in the shape of doctrines of Paramarthika and Vyavaharika. (V. 15.)

13. The one great cause of the downfall and the degeneration of India was the building of a wall of custom—whose foundation was hatred of others—round the nation, and the real aim of which in ancient times was to prevent the Hindus from coming in contact with the surrounding Buddhistic nations. Whatever cloak ancient or modern sophistry may try to throw over it, the inevitable result—the vindication of the moral law that none can hate others without

degenerating himself—is that the race that was foremost amongst the ancient races is now a byword, and a scorn among nations. We are the object lessons of the violation of that law which our ancestors were the first to discover and disseminate. (IV. 365.)

XXVI

INDIA—Her Characteristics

1. The debt which the world owes to our Motherland is immense. Taking country with country, there is not one race on this earth to which the world owes so much as to the patient Hindu, the mild Hindu. (III. 105.)

2. Those who keep their eyes open, those who understand the workings in the minds of the different nations of the West, those who are thinkers and study the different nations, will find the immense change that has been produced in the tone, the procedure, in the methods, and in the literature of the world by this slow, never-ceasing permeation of Indian thought. (III. 109.)

3. Each race has a peculiar bent, each race has a peculiar *raison d'être*, each race has a peculiar mission to fulfil in the life of the world. Each race has to make its own result, to fulfil its own mission. Political greatness or military power is never the mission of our race; it never was, and, mark my words, it never will be. But there has been the other mission given to us, which is to conserve, to preserve, to accumulate, as it were, into a dynamo, all the spiritual energy of the race, and that concentrated energy is to

INDIA—HER CHARACTERISTICS

pour forth in a deluge on the world, whenever circumstances are propitious. (III. 108-09.)

4. India's gift to the world is the light spiritual. (III. 109.)

5. Religious researches disclose to us the fact that there is not a country possessing a good ethical code but has borrowed something of it from us, and there is not one religion possessing good ideas of the immortality of the soul but has derived it directly or indirectly from us. (III. 138.)

6. Gifts of political knowledge can be made with the blasts of trumpets and the march of cohorts. Gifts of secular knowledge and social knowledge can be made with fire and sword; but spiritual knowledge can only be given in silence, like the dew that falls unseen and unheard, yet bringing into bloom masses of roses. This has been the gift of India to the world again and again. (III. 222.)

7. Whenever there has been a great conquering race, bringing the nations of the world together, making roads and transit possible, immediately India arose and gave her quota of spiritual power to the sum total of the progress of the world. (III. 222.)

8. Like the gentle dew that falls unseen and unheard, and yet brings into blossom the fairest of roses, has been the contribution of India to

the thought of the world. Silent, unperceived, yet omnipotent in its effect, it has revolutionised the thought of the world, yet nobody knows when it did so. (III. 274.)

9. The one characteristic of Indian thought is its silence, its calmness. At the same time the tremendous power that is behind it is never expressed by violence. (III. 274.)

10. I challenge anybody to show one single period of her national life when India was lacking in spiritual giants, capable of moving the world. (IV. 315.)

11. In this land are, still, religion and spirituality, the fountains which will have to overflow and flood the world, to bring in new life and new vitality to the Western and other nations, which are now almost borne down, half-killed and degraded by political ambitions and social scheming. (III. 148.)

12. Shall India die? Then from the world all spirituality will be extinct; all moral perfection will be extinct; all sweet-souled sympathy for religion will be extinct; all ideality will be extinct; and in its place will reign the duality of lust and luxury as the male and female deities, with money as its priest; fraud, force and competition its ceremonies; and the human soul its sacrifice. Such a thing can never be. The power of suffering is infinitely greater than the power

of doing; the power of love is infinitely of greater potency than the power of hatred. (IV. 348.)

13. There may be people whose brains have become turned by the Western luxurious ideals; there may be thousands and hundreds of thousands, who have drunk deep of enjoyment, this curse of the West, the senses, the curse of the world, yet for all that, there will be other thousands in this motherland of mine to whom religion will be a reality, and who will be ever ready to give up without counting the cost, if need be. (III. 345.)

14. This is the theme of Indian life-work, the burden of her eternal songs, the *raison d'être* of her very existence—the spiritualisation of the human race. In this her life-course she has never deviated, whether the Tartar ruled or the Turk, whether the Mogul ruled or the English. (IV. 315.)

15. Our method is very easily described. It simply consists in reasserting the national life. ... The secret lies there. The national ideals of India are RENUNCIATION and SERVICE. Intensify her in those channels, and the rest will take care of itself. The banner of the spiritual cannot be raised too high in this country. In it alone is salvation. (V. 228.)

16. Our sacred motherland is the land of religion and philosophy—the birthplace of spirit-

ual giants—the land of renunciation, where and where alone, from the most ancient to the most modern times, there has been the highest ideal of life open to man. (III. 137.)

17. This is the motherland of philosophy, of spirituality, and of ethics, of sweetness, gentleness, and love.... India is still the first and foremost of all the nations of the world in these respects. (III. 147.)

XXVII

INDIA—THE WAY TO HER REGENERATION

1. We talk foolishly against material civilisation. The grapes are sour. Even taking all that foolishness for granted, in all India there are, say, a hundred thousand really spiritual men and women. Now, for the spiritualisation of these, must three hundred millions be sunk in savagery and starvation? Why should they starve? How was it possible for the Hindus to have been conquered by the Mohammedans? It was due to the Hindus' ignorance of material civilisation.... Material civilisation, nay even luxury, is necessary to create work for the poor. Bread! Bread! I do not believe in a God who cannot give me bread here, giving me eternal bliss in heaven! Pooh! India is to be raised, the poor are to be fed, education is to be spread, and the evil of priestcraft is to be removed. No priestcraft, no social tyranny! More bread, more opportunity for everybody! ...

Now, this is to be brought about slowly and by only insisting on our religion, and giving liberty to society. Root up priestcraft from the old religion and you get the best religion in the world. Do you understand me? Can you make a

European society with India's religion? I believe it is possible and must be. (IV. 368.)

2. The country has fallen, no doubt, but will as surely rise again, and that upheaval will astound the world. The lower the hollows the billows make, the higher and with equal force will they rise again. (V. 381.)

3. You all set your shoulders to the wheel! ... Your duty at present is to go from one part of the country to another, from village to village, and make the people understand that mere sitting about idly won't do any more. Make them understand their real condition and say, "O ye brothers, all arise! Awake! How much longer would you remain asleep!" Go and advise them how to improve their own condition, and make them comprehend the sublime truths of the Scriptures, by presenting them in a lucid and popular way.... Also instruct them, in simple words, about the necessities of life, and in trade, commerce, agriculture, etc. If you cannot do this, then fie upon your education and culture, and fie upon your studying the Vedas and Vedanta! (V. 381.)

4. Religion for a long time has come to be static in India. What we want is to make it dynamic. I want it to be brought into the life of everybody. Religion, as it always has been in the past, must enter the palaces of kings as

INDIA—THE WAY TO HER REGENERATION 163

well as the homes of the poorest peasants in the land. Religion, the common inheritance, the universal birthright of the race, must be brought free to the door of everybody. Religion in India must be made as free and as easy of access as is God's air. And this is the kind of work we have to bring about in India, but not by getting up little sects and fighting on points of difference. Let us preach where we all agree, and leave the differences to remedy themselves. As I have said ... again and again, if there is the darkness of centuries in a room, and we go into the room and begin to cry, "Oh, it is dark, it is dark!" will the darkness go? Bring in the light and the darkness will vanish at once. (III. 383.)

5. Take care of these two things—love of power and jealousy. Cultivate always faith in yourself. (V. 52.)

6. First go to other countries and study carefully their manners and conditions with your own eyes—not with others'—and reflect on them ... then read your own Scriptures, your ancient literature, travel throughout India and mark the people of her different parts and their ways and habits with the wide-awake eye of an intelligent and keen observer ... and you will see as clean as noonday that the nation is still living intact and its life is surely pulsating. You will find there, also, that hidden under the ashes of

apparent death, the fire of our national life is yet smouldering and that the life of this nation is religion, its language religion and its idea religion; and your politics, society, municipality, plague-prevention work and famine-relief work —all these things will be done as they have been done all along here, viz only through religion; otherwise all your frantic yelling and bewailing will end in nothing, my friend! (V. 460-61.)

7. We cannot do without the world outside India; it was our foolishness that we thought we could, and we have paid the penalty by about a thousand years of slavery. That we did not go out to compare things with other nations, did not mark the workings that have been all around us, has been the one great cause of this degradation of the Indian mind. We have paid the penalty; let us do it no more. (III. 272.)

8. We have to learn from others. You put the seed in the ground, and give it plenty of earth, and air, and water to feed upon; when the seed grows into the plant, and into a gigantic tree, does it become the earth, does it become the air, or does it become the water? It becomes the mighty plant, the mighty tree, after its own nature, having absorbed everything that was given to it. Let that be your position. We have indeed many things to learn from others, yea,

that man who refuses to learn is already dead. (III. 381.)

9. A hundred thousand men and women, fired with the zeal of holiness, fortified with eternal faith in the Lord, and nerved to lion's courage by their sympathy for the poor and the fallen and the downtrodden, will go over the length and breadth of the land, preaching the gospel of salvation, the gospel of help, the gospel of social raising-up—the gospel of equality. (V. 15.)

10. The hope lies in you—in the meek, the lowly but the faithful. Have faith in the Lord; no policy, it is nothing. Feel for the miserable and look up for help—it *shall come*. I have travelled twelve years with this load in my heart and this idea in my head. I have gone from door to door of the so-called rich and great. With a bleeding heart I have crossed half the world to this strange land, seeking for help. The Lord is great. I know He will help me. I may perish of cold or hunger in this land, but I bequeath to you, young men, this sympathy, this struggle for the poor, the ignorant, the oppressed. Go now this minute to the temple of Parthasarathi, and before Him who was friend to the poor and the lowly cowherds of Gokula, who never shrank to embrace the Pariah Guhaka, who accepted the invitation of a prostitute in preference to that of the nobles and saved her in His incarnation as

Buddha—yea, down on your faces before Him, and make a great sacrifice, the sacrifice of a whole life for them, for whom He comes from time to time, whom He loves above all, the poor, the lowly, the oppressed. Vow, then, to devote your whole lives to the cause of the redemption of these three hundred millions, going down and down every day. (V. 16-17.)

11. Then only will India awake, when hundreds of large-hearted men and women giving up all desires of enjoying the luxuries of life, will long and exert themselves to their utmost for the well-being of the millions of their countrymen who are gradually sinking lower and lower in the vortex of destitution and ignorance. I have experienced even in my insignificant life that good motives, sincerity and infinite love can conquer the world. One single soul possessed of these virtues can destroy the dark designs of millions of hypocrites and brutes. (V. 127.)

12. You merge yourselves in the void and disappear, and let New India arise in your place. Let her arise—out of the peasants' cottage, grasping the plough, out of the huts of the fisherman, the cobbler and the sweeper. Let her spring from the grocer's shop, from beside the oven of the fritter-seller. Let her emanate from the factory, from marts and from markets. Let her emerge from the groves and forests, from

hills and mountains. These common people have suffered oppression for thousands of years—suffered it without murmur, and as a result have got wonderful fortitude. They have suffered eternal misery, which has given them unflinching vitality. Living on a handful of oatmeal they can convulse the world; give them only half a piece of bread, and the whole world will not be big enough to contain their energy; they are endowed with the inexhaustible vitality of a Raktabija[1]. And, besides, they have got the wonderful strength that comes of a pure and moral life, which is not to be found anywhere else in the world. Such peacefulness, such contentment, such love, such power of silent and incessant work, and such manifestation of lion's strength in times of action—where else will you find these! Skeletons of the past, there, before you, are your successors, the India that is to be. Throw those treasure-chests of yours and those jewelled rings among them—as soon as you can; and you—vanish into air, and be seen no more—only keep your eyes open: No sooner will you disappear than you will hear the inaugural shout of Renaissant India—ringing with the voice of a million thunders and reverberating throughout

---

[1] A powerful demon mentioned in the *Durga Saptashati*, every drop of whose blood produced another demon like him.

the universe—"Wah Guru Ki Fateh—Victory to the Guru!" (VII. 327-28.)

13. Give up this filthy Vamachara that is killing your country. You have not seen the other parts of India. When I see how much the Vamachara has entered our society, I find it a most disgraceful place with all its boast of culture. These Vamachara sects are honeycombing our society in Bengal. Those who come out in the day-time and preach most loudly about Āchara, it is they who carry on the horrible debauchery at night and are backed by the most dreadful books. They are ordered by the books to do these things. You who are of Bengal know it. The Bengali Shastras are the Vamachara Tantras. They are published by the cartload, and you poison the minds of your children with them instead of teaching them your shrutis. Fathers of Calcutta, do you not feel ashamed that such horrible stuff as these Vamachara Tantras, with translations too, should be put into the hands of your boys and girls, and their minds poisoned, and that they should be brought up with the idea that these are the Shastras of the Hindus? If you are ashamed, take them away from your children, and let them read the true Shastras, the Vedas, the Gita, the Upanishads. (III. 340-41.)

14. Can you adduce any reason why India

should lie in the ebb-tide of the Aryan nations? Is she inferior in intellect? Is she inferior in dexterity? Can you look at her art, at her mathematics, at her philosophy, and answer "yes"? All that is needed is that she should dehypnotise herself and wake up from her age-long sleep to take her true rank in the hierarchy of nations. (V. 227.)

15. Now is wanted—as said in the Gita by the Lord—intense Karma-Yoga, with unbounded courage and indomitable strength in the heart. Then only will the people of the country be roused, otherwise they will continue to be as much in the dark as you are. (VII. 185.)

16. Do you know what my idea is? By preaching the profound secrets of the Vedanta religion in the Western world, we shall attract the sympathy and regard of these mighty nations, maintaining for ever the position of their teacher in spiritual matters, and they will remain our teachers in all material concerns. ... Nothing will come of crying day and night before them, "Give me this or give me that". When there will grow a link of sympathy and regard between both nations by this give-and-take intercourse, there will be then no need for these noisy cries. They will do everything of their own accord. I believe that by this cultivation of religion and the wider diffusion of the Vedanta, both this

country and the West will gain enormously. To me the pursuit of politics is a secondary means in comparison with this. I will lay down my life to carry out this belief practically. If you believe in any other way of accomplishing the good of India, well, you may go on working your own way. (VI. 448-49.)

17. None will be able to resist truth and love and sincerity. Are you sincere? unselfish even unto death? and loving? Then fear not, not even death. Onward, my lads! The whole world requires Light. It is expectant! India alone has that Light, not in magic mummeries and charlatanism, but in the teaching of the glories of the spirit of real religion—of the highest spiritual truth. That is why the Lord has preserved the race through all its vicissitudes unto the present day. Now the time has come. Have faith that you are all, my brave lads, born to do great things! Let not the barks of puppies frighten you—no, not even the thunderbolts of heaven—but stand up and work! (V. 43.)

18. My whole ambition in life is to set in motion a machinery which will bring noble ideas to the door of everybody, and then let men and women settle their own fate. Let them know what our forefathers as well as other nations have thought on the most momentous questions of life. Let them see specially what others are

doing now, and then decide. We are to put the chemicals together, the crystallisation will be done by nature according to her laws. Work hard, be steady, and have faith in the Lord. Set to work, I am coming sooner or later. Keep the motto before you—"Elevation of the masses without injuring their religion".

Remember that the nation lives in the cottage. But, alas! nobody ever did anything for them. Our modern reformers are very busy about widow remarriage. Of course, I am a sympathiser in every reform, but the fate of a nation does not depend upon the number of husbands their widows get, but upon the *condition of the masses*. Can you raise them? Can you give them back their lost individuality without making them lose their innate spiritual nature? Can you become an occidental of occidentals in your spirit of equality, freedom, work, and energy, and at the same time a Hindu to the very backbone in religious culture and instincts? This is to be done and *we will do it*. You are all *born to do it*. Have faith in yourselves, great convictions are the mothers of great deeds. Onward for ever! Sympathy for the poor, the downtrodden, even unto death—this is our motto. (V. 29-30.)

19. Now is needed the worship of Sri Krishna uttering forth the lion-roar of the Gita, of Rama with His bow and arrows, of Mahavira, of

Mother Kali. Then only will the people grow strong by going to work with great energy and will. I have considered the matter most carefully and come to the conclusion that of those who profess and talk of religion nowadays in this country, the majority are full of morbidity—crack-brained or fanatic. Without the development of an abundance of Rajas (activity), you have hopes neither in this world, nor in the next. The whole country is enveloped in intense Tamas (inertia); and naturally the result is—servitude in this life and hell in the next. (VI. 458.)

20. Be patriots, love the race which has done such great things in the past. Ay, the more I compare notes the more I love you, my fellow-countrymen; you are good and pure and gentle. You have always been tyrannised over, and such is the irony of this material world of Maya. Never mind that; the spirit will triumph in the long run. In the meanwhile let us work and let us not abuse our country, let us not curse and abuse the weather-beaten and work-worn institutions of our thrice-holy motherland. (III. 199.)

XXVIII

KRISHNA AND KARMA-YOGA

1. He (Krishna) is the most rounded man I know of, wonderfully developed equally in brain and heart and hand. Every moment (of his) is alive with activity, either as a gentleman, warrior, minister, or something else. Great as a gentleman, as a scholar, as a poet. This all-rounded and wonderful activity and combination of brain and heart you see in the Gita and other books. Most wonderful heart, exquisite language, and nothing can approach it anywhere. This tremendous activity of the man—the impression is still there. Five thousand years have passed and he has influenced millions and millions. Just think what an influence this man has over the whole world, whether you know it or not. My regard for him is for his perfect sanity. No cobwebs in that brain, no superstition. He knows the use of everything, and when it is necessary to (assign a place to each), he is there. (I. 457.)

2. This was the great work of Krishna: To clear our eyes and make us look with broader vision upon humanity in its march upward and onward. His was the first heart that was large enough to see truth in all, his the first lips that uttered beautiful words for each and all. (I. 438.)

3. Two ideas (stand) supreme in his message: The first is the harmony of different ideas; the second is non-attachment. (I. 438.)

4. A great landmark in the history of religion is here, the ideal of love for love's sake, work for work's sake, duty for duty's sake, and it for the first time fell from the lips of the greatest of Incarnations, Krishna, and for the first time in the history of humanity, upon the soil of India. The religions of fear and of temptations were gone for ever, and in spite of the fear of hell, and temptation of enjoyment in heaven, came the grandest of ideals, love for love's sake, duty for duty's sake, work for work's sake. (III. 258.)

5. Every one must work in the universe. Only those who are perfectly satisfied with the Self, whose desires do not go beyond the Self, whose mind never strays out of the Self, to whom the Self is all in all, only those do not work. The rest must work. (I. 98.)

6. Although a man has not studied a single system of philosophy, although he does not believe in any God, and never has believed, although he has not prayed even once in his life, if the simple power of good actions has brought him to that state where he is ready to give up his life and all else for others, he has arrived at the same point to which the religious man will come through his prayers and the philosopher

through his knowledge; and so you may find that the philosopher, the worker, and the devotee, all meet at one point, that one point being self-abnegation. However much their systems of philosophy and religion may differ, all mankind stand in reverence and awe before the man who is ready to sacrifice himself for others. (I. 86.)

7. According to Karma-Yoga, the action one has done cannot be destroyed, until it has borne its fruit; no power in nature can stop it from yielding its results. If I do an evil action, I must suffer for it; there is no power in this universe to stop it or stay it. Similarly, if I do a good action, there is no power in the universe which can stop its bearing good results. The cause must have its effect; nothing can prevent or restrain this. (I. 82.)

8. Law is the method, the manner in which our mind grasps a series of phenomena; it is all in the mind. Certain phenomena, happening one after another or together, and followed by the conviction of the regularity of their recurrence, thus enabling our minds to grasp the method of the whole series constitute what we call law. (I. 95.)

9. The ideal man is he who, in the midst of the greatest silence and solitude, finds the intensest activity, and in the midst of the intensest activity finds the silence and solitude of the

desert. He has learned the secret of restraint, he has controlled himself. He goes through the streets of a big city with all its traffic, and his mind is as calm as if he were in a cave, where not a sound could reach him; and he is intensely working all the time. That is the ideal of Karma-Yoga, and if you have attained to that you have really learned the secret of work. (I. 34.)

10. Now you see what Karma-Yoga means; even at the point of death to help any one, without asking questions. Be cheated millions of times and never ask a question, and never think of what you are doing. Never vaunt of your gifts to the poor or expect their gratitude, but rather be grateful to them for giving you the occasion of practising charity to them. (I. 62.)

11. What is Karma-Yoga? The knowledge of the secret of work.... Instead of being knocked about in this universe, and after long delay and thrashing, getting to know things as they are, we learn from Karma-Yoga the secret of work, the method of work, the organising power of work. A vast mass of energy may be spent in vain, if we do not know how to utilise it. Karma-Yoga makes a science of work, you learn by it how best to utilise all the working of this world. Work is inevitable, it must be so; but we should work to the highest purpose. (I. 99.)

12. "Work incessantly, but give up all

attachment to work." Do not identify yourself with anything. Hold your mind free. All this that you see, the pains and miseries are but the necessary conditions of this world; poverty and wealth and happiness are but momentary; they do not belong to our real nature at all. Our nature is far beyond misery and happiness, beyond every object of the senses, beyond the imagination; and yet we must go on working all the time. "Misery comes through attachment, not through work." As soon as we identify ourselves with the work we do, we feel miserable; but if we do not identify ourselves with it we do not feel that misery. (I. 100.)

13. This "I and mine" causes the whole misery. With the sense of possession comes selfishness, and selfishness brings on misery. Every act of selfishness or thought of selfishness makes us attached to something, and immediately we are made slaves. Each wave in the Chitta that says "I and mine", immediately puts a chain round us and makes us slaves; and the more we say "I and mine", the more slavery grows, the more misery increases. Therefore, Karma-Yoga tells us to enjoy the beauty of all the pictures in the world but not to identify ourselves with any of them. (I. 100.)

14. So Karma-Yoga says, first destroy the tendency to project this tentacle of selfishness,

and when you have the power of checking it, hold it in and do not allow the mind to get into the ways of selfishness. Then you may go out into the world and work as much as you can. Mix everywhere; go where you please; you will never be contaminated with evil. There is the lotus leaf in the water; the water cannot touch and adhere to it; so will you be in the world. (I. 101.)

15. Non-attachment does not mean anything that we may do in relation to our external body, it is all in the mind. The binding link of "I and mine" is in the mind. If we have not this link with the body and with the things of the senses, we are non-attached, wherever and whatever we may be. A man may be on the throne and perfectly non-attached; another man may be in rags and still very attached. First, we have to attain this state of non-attachment, and then to work incessantly. Karma-Yoga gives us the method that will help us in giving up all attachment, though it is very hard. (I. 101-02.)

16. Here are two ways of giving up all attachment. The one is for those who do not believe in God, or in any outside help. They are left to their own devices; they have simply to work with their own will, with the powers of their mind and discrimination, saying, "I must be non-attached". For those who believe in God there

KRISHNA AND KARMA-YOGA 179

is another way, which is much less difficult. They give up the fruits of work unto the Lord, they work and are never attached to the results. Whatever they see, feel, hear, or do, is for Him. For whatever good work we may do, let us not claim any praise or benefit. It is the Lord's; give up the fruits unto Him. (I. 102.)

17. Instead of the sacrifice of pouring oblations into the fire, perform this one great sacrifice day and night—the sacrifice of your little self. "In search of wealth in this world, Thou art the only wealth I have found; I sacrifice myself unto Thee." Let us repeat this day and night, and say, "Nothing for me; no matter whether the thing is good, bad, or indifferent; I do not care for it; I sacrifice all unto Thee". Day and night let us renounce our seeming self until it becomes a habit with us to do so, until it gets into the blood, the nerves and the brain, and the whole body is every moment obedient to this idea of self-renunciation. Go then into the midst of the battlefield, with the roaring cannon and the din of war, and you will find yourself to be free and at peace. (I. 102.)

18. I want to do work, I want to do good to a human being; and it is ninety to one that that human being whom I have helped will prove ungrateful, and go against me; and the result to me is pain. Such things deter mankind from

working; and it spoils a good portion of the work and energy of mankind, this fear of pain and misery. Karma-Yoga teaches us how to work for work's sake, unattached, without caring who is helped, and what for. The Karma-Yogi works because it is his nature, because he *feels* that it is good for him to do so, and he has no object beyond that. His position in this world is that of a giver, and he never cares to receive anything. He knows that he is giving, and does not ask for anything in return and therefore he eludes the grasp of misery. (II. 392.)

19. Karma-Yoga is the attainment through unselfish work of that freedom which is the goal of all human nature. Every selfish action, therefore, retards our reaching the goal, and every unselfish action takes us towards the goal; that is why the only definition that can be given of morality is this—*That which is selfish is immoral, and that which is unselfish is moral.* (I. 110.)

20. The Karma-Yogi need not believe in any doctrine whatever. He may not believe even in God, may not ask what his soul is, nor think of any metaphysical speculation. He has got his own special aim of realising selflessness; and he has to work it out himself. Every moment of his life must be realisation because he has to solve by mere work, without the help of doctrine or theory, the very same problem to which the

KRISHNA AND KARMA-YOGA 181

Jnani applies his reason and inspiration and the Bhakta his love. (I. 111.)

21. Plunge into the world and learn the secret of work, and that is the way of Karma-Yoga. Do not fly away from the wheels of the world-machine, but stand inside it and learn the secret of work. Through proper work done inside, it is possible to come out. Through this machinery itself is the way out. (I. 115.)

22. I have been asked many times how we can work if we do not have the passion which we generally feel for work. I also thought in that way years ago, but as I am growing older, getting more experience, I find it is not true. The less passion there is, the better we work. The calmer we are, the better for us, and the more the amount of work we can do. When we let loose our feelings we waste so much energy, shatter our nerves, disturb our minds, and accomplish very little work. The energy which ought to have gone out as work is spent as mere feeling, which counts for nothing. It is only when the mind is very calm and collected that the whole of its energy is spent in doing good work. And if you read the lives of the great workers which the world has produced, you will find that they were wonderfully calm men. Nothing, as it were, could throw them off their balance. That is why the man who becomes angry never does a great

amount of work, and the man whom nothing can make angry accomplishes so much. The man who gives way to anger, or hatred, or any other passion, cannot work, he only breaks himself to pieces, and does nothing practical. It is the calm, forgiving, equable, well-balanced mind that does the greatest amount of work. (II. 293.)

23. A man ought to live in this world like a lotus leaf, which grows in water but is never moistened by water; so a man ought to live in the world—his heart to God and his hands to work. (I. 12.)

24. Talk does not count for anything. Parrots can do that. Perfection comes through the disinterested performance of action. (IV. 137.)

25. Swamiji: True, power comes of austerities; but again, working for the sake of others itself constitutes Tapasya (practice of austerity). The Karma-Yogis regard work itself as a part of Tapasya. As on the one hand the practice of Tapasya intensifies altruistic feelings in the devotee and actuates him to unselfish work, so also the pursuit of work for the sake of others carries the worker to the last fruition of Tapasya, namely, the purification of the heart, and leads him thus to the realisation of the supreme Atman.

Disciple: But, sir, how few of us can work whole-heartedly for the sake of others from the very outset! How difficult it is for such

KRISHNA AND KARMA-YOGA 185

driven about by every circumstance, ordered about by the laws of nature, drifting from place to place. That would be the result. But that is not what is meant. We must work. Ordinary mankind, driven everywhere by false desire, what do they know of work? The man propelled by his own feelings and his own senses, what does he know about work? He works, who is not propelled by his own desires, by any selfishness whatsoever. He works, who has no ulterior motive in view. He works, who has nothing to gain from work. (II. 148-49.)

XXIX

KNOWLEDGE AND IGNORANCE

1. You are pure already, you are free already. If you think you are free, free you are this moment; and if you think you are bound, bound you will be. This is a very bold statement.... It may frighten you now, but when you think over it, and realise it in your own life, then you will come to know that what I say is true. For, supposing that freedom is not your nature, by no manner of means can you become free. Supposing you were free and in some way you lost that freedom, that shows that you were not free to begin with. Had you been free, what could have made you lose it? (II. 195-96.)

2. Various clouds of various colours come before the sky. They remain there a minute and then pass away. It is the cloud that is changing. So you are always perfect, eternally perfect. Nothing ever changes your nature, or ever will. All these ideas that I am imperfect, I am a man, or a woman, or a sinner, or I am the mind, I have thought, I will think, all are hallucinations; you never think, you never had a body; you never were imperfect. (III. 9.)

3. You are in all, and you are all. Whom to avoid, and whom to take? You are the all in all.

When this knowledge comes, delusion immediately vanishes. (III. 9.)

4. Place, time, causation are all delusions. It is your disease that you think you are bound and will be free. You are the unchangeable. Talk not. Sit down and let all things melt away, they are but dreams. There is no differentiation, no distinction, it is all superstition; therefore be silent and know what you are. (VII. 73-74.)

5. Fear naught, you are the essence of existence. Be at peace. Do not disturb yourself. You never were in bondage, you never were virtuous or sinful. Get rid of all these delusions and be at peace.... All is the Atman. To speak, to think is superstition. Repeat over and over, "I am Atman", "I am Atman". Let everything else go. (VII. 74.)

6. Ignorance is the cause of all this bondage. It is through ignorance that we have become bound; knowledge will cure it, by taking us to the other side. How will that knowledge come? Through love, Bhakti. By the worship of God, by loving all beings as the temples of God; He resides within them. Thus, with that intense love will come knowledge and ignorance will disappear, the bonds will break, and the soul will be free. (III. 128.)

7. To get any reason out of the mass of incongruity we call human life, we have to

transcend our reason, but we must do it scientifically, slowly, by regular practice, and we must cast off all superstition. We must take up the study of the superconscious state just as any other science. On reason we must have to lay our foundation, we must follow reason as far as it leads, and when reason fails, reason itself will show us the way to the highest plane. (I. 184-85.)

8. The great question of all questions at the present time is this: Taking for granted that the known and the knowable are bounded on both sides by the unknowable and the infinitely unknown, why struggle for that infinite unknown? Why shall we not be content with the known? Why shall we not rest satisfied with eating, drinking, and doing a little good to society? This idea is in the air. From the most learned professor to the prattling baby, we are told to do good to the world, that is all of religion, and that it is useless to trouble ourselves about questions of the beyond. So much is this the case that it has become a truism.

But fortunately we *must* inquire into the beyond. This present, this expressed, is only one part of that unexpressed. The sense universe is, as it were, only one portion, one bit of that infinite spiritual universe projected into the plane of sense consciousness. How can this little bit

KNOWLEDGE AND IGNORANCE

of projection be explained, be understood, without knowing that which is beyond? (III. 2.)

9. Kant has proved beyond all doubt that we cannot penetrate beyond the tremendous dead wall called reason. But that is the very first idea upon which all Indian thought takes its stand, and dares to seek, and succeeds in finding something higher than reason, where alone the explanation of the present state is found. This is the value of the study of something that will take us beyond the world. "Thou art our father, and wilt take us to the other shore of this ocean of ignorance." That is the science of religion, nothing else. (I. 199.)

10. Why religions should claim that they are not bound to abide by the standpoint of reason, no one knows. If one does not take the standard of reason there cannot be any true judgment, even in the case of religions. One religion may ordain something very hideous. For instance, the Mohammedan religion allows Mohammedans to kill all who are not of their religion. It is clearly stated in the Koran, "Kill the infidels if they do not become Mohammedans". They must be put to fire and sword. Now if we tell a Mohammedan that this is wrong, he will naturally ask: "How do you know that? How do you know it is not good? My book says it is." If you say your book is older, there will come the Buddhist,

and say, his book is much older still. Then will come the Hindu, and say, his books are the oldest of all. Therefore referring to books will not do. Where is the standard by which you can compare? You will say, look at the Sermon on the Mount, and the Mohammedan will reply, look at the Ethics of the Koran. The Mohammedan will say, who is the arbiter as to which is the better of the two? Neither the New Testament nor the Koran can be the arbiter in a quarrel between them. There must be some independent authority, and that cannot be any book, but something which is universal; and what is more universal than reason? It has been said that reason is not strong enough; it does not always help us to get the Truth; many times it makes mistakes, and therefore the conclusion is that we must believe in the authority of a church! That was said to me by a Roman Catholic, but I could not see the logic of it. On the other hand I should say, if reason be so weak, a body of priests would be weaker, and I am not going to accept their verdict but I will abide by my reason, because with all its weakness there is some chance of my getting at truth through it; while by the other means, there is no such hope at all. (II. 335-36.)

11. Then arises the question, how can all these varieties be true? If one thing is true, its negation is false. How can contradictory opinions be true

KNOWLEDGE AND IGNORANCE

at the same time? This is the question which I intend to answer. But I will first ask you: Are all the religions of the world really contradictory? I do not mean the external forms in which great thoughts are clad. I do not mean the different buildings, languages, rituals, books, etc., employed in various religions, but I mean the internal soul of every religion. Every religion has a soul behind it, and that soul may differ from the soul of another religion; but are they contradictory? Do they contradict or supplement each other—that is the question. I took up the question when I was quite a boy, and have been studying it all my life. Thinking that my conclusion may be of some help to you, I place it before you. I believe that they are not contradictory; they are supplementary. Each religion, as it were, takes up one part of the great universal truth, and spends its whole force in embodying and typifying that part of the great truth. It is therefore addition, not exclusion. That is the idea. System after system arises, each one embodying a great idea, and ideals must be added to ideals. And this is the march of humanity. Man never progresses from error to truth, but from truth to truth, from lesser truth to higher truth—but it is never from error to truth. (II. 365.)

XXX

MAN

1. This human body is the greatest body in the universe, and a human being the greatest being. Man is higher than all animals, than all angels; none is greater than man. Even the Devas (gods) will have to come down again and attain to perfection through a human body. Man alone attains to perfection, not even the Devas. According to the Jews and Mohammedans, God created man after creating the angels and everything else, and after creating man He asked the angels to come and salute him, and all did so except Iblis; so God cursed him and he became Satan. Behind the allegory is the great truth that this human birth is the greatest birth we can have. (I. 142.)

2. It is a significant fact that all religions, without one exception, hold that man is a degeneration of what he was, whether they clothe this in mythological words, or in the clear language of philosophy, or in the beautiful expressions of poetry. (II. 272.)

3. The Real Man is one and infinite, the omnipresent spirit. And the apparent man, however great he may be, is only a dim reflection of the Real Man, who is beyond. The Real Man,

the Spirit, being beyond cause and effect, not bound by time and space, must therefore be free.... The apparent man, the reflection, is limited by time, space, and causation, and is therefore bound. Or in the language of some of our philosophers, he appears to be bound, but really is not. (II. 78.)

4. No books, no scriptures, no science can ever imagine the glory of the Self that appears as man, the most glorious God that ever was, the only God that ever existed, exists, or ever will exist. (II. 250.)

5. Man, after his vain search after various gods outside himself, completes the circle, and comes back to the point from which he started— the human soul, and he finds that the God whom he was searching in hill and dale, whom he was seeking in every brook, in every temple, in churches and heavens, that God whom he was imagining as sitting in heaven and ruling the world, is his own Self. I am He, and He is I. None but I was God, and this little I never existed. (II. 250-51.)

6. You may invent an image through which to worship God, but a better image already exists, the living man. You may build a temple in which to worship God, and that may be good, but a better one, a much higher one, already exists, the human body. (II. 313.)

7. The living God is within you, and yet you are building churches and temples and believing all sorts of imaginary nonsense. The only God to worship is the human soul in the human body. Of course all animals are temples too, but man is the highest, the Taj Mahal of temples. If I cannot worship in that, no other temple will be of any advantage. The moment I have realised God sitting in the temple of every human body, the moment I stand in reverence before every human being and see God in him—that moment I am free from bondage, everything that binds vanishes, and I am free. (II. 321.)

8. When a man has no more self in him, no possession, nothing to call "me" or "mine", has given himself up entirely, destroyed himself as it were—in that man is God Himself; for in him self-will is gone, crushed out, annihilated. That is the ideal man. (IV. 150.)

9. The growth of man can only be gauged by his power of living in the higher atmosphere where the senses are left behind, the amount of the pure thought-oxygen his lungs can breathe in, and the amount of time he can spend on that height. (IV. 284.)

10. First, let us be Gods, and then help others to be Gods. "Be and make." Let this be our motto. Say not man is a sinner. Tell him that he is a God. Even if there were a devil, it would

be our duty to remember God always and not the devil. (IV. 351.)

11. When you think you are a body, you are apart from the universe; when you think you are a soul, you are a spark from the great Eternal Fire; when you think you are the Atman, you are All. (V. 409.)

12. No great work can be achieved by humbug. It is through Love, a passion for Truth, and tremendous energy, that all undertakings are accomplished. तत् कुरु पौरुषम्—Therefore, manifest your manhood. (VI. 330.)

13. It is not law that we want, but the ability to break law. We want to be outlaws. If you are bound by laws, you will be a lump of clay. Whether you are beyond the law or not is not the question; but the thought that we are beyond law—upon that is based the whole history of humanity. (V. 289.)

14. Each man is the Infinite already, only these bars and bolts and different circumstances shut him in, but as soon as they are removed, he rushes out and expresses himself. (V. 298.)

15. Every man is a slave except the Yogi. He is a slave to food, to air, to his wife, to his children, to a dollar, slave to a nation, slave to name and fame, and to a thousand things in the world. The man who is not controlled by any

one of these bondages is alone a real man, a real Yogi. (V. 305.)

16. Every one has an opportunity within the limits of his present development of making himself better. We cannot unmake ourselves; we cannot destroy or impair the vital force within us, but we have the freedom to give it different directions. (V. 312.)

17. Men should be taught to be practical and physically strong. A dozen of such lions will conquer the world, and not millions of sheep can do so. Secondly, men should not be taught to imitate a personal ideal, however great. (V. 315.)

18. Man is like an infinite spring, coiled up in a small box, and the spring is trying to unfold itself; and all the social phenomena that we see are the result of this trying to unfold. (I. 389.)

19. Ye are the Children of God, the sharers of immortal bliss, holy and perfect beings. Ye divinities on earth—sinners! It is a sin to call a man so; it is a standing libel on human nature. (I. 11.)

20. Each one of us has come out of one protoplasmic cell, and all the powers we possess were coiled up there.... The energy was there, potentially no doubt, but still there. So is infinite power in the soul of man, whether he knows it or not. Its manifestation is only a question of being conscious of it. Slowly this infinite giant

is, as it were, waking up, becoming conscious of his power, and arousing himself; and with his growing consciousness, more and more of his bonds are breaking, chains are bursting asunder, and the day is sure to come when, with the full consciousness of his infinite power and wisdom, the giant will rise to his feet and stand erect. Let us all help to hasten that glorious consummation. (II. 340.)

XXXI

MAYA

1. When the Hindu says the world is Maya, at once people get the idea that the world is an illusion. This interpretation has some basis, as coming through the Buddhistic philosophers, because there was one section of philosophers who did not believe in the external world at all. But the Maya of Vedanta, in its last developed form is neither Idealism nor Realism, nor is it a theory. It is a simple statement of facts—what we are, and what we see around us. (II. 89.)

2. The one peculiar attribute we find in time, space, and causation is that they cannot exist separate from other things. Try to think of space without colour, or limits, or any connection with the things around—just abstract space. You cannot; you have to think of it as the space between two limits, or between three objects. It has to be connected with some object to have any existence. So with time; you cannot have any idea of abstract time, but you have to take two events, one preceding, and the other succeeding, and join the two events by the idea of succession. Time depends on two events, just as space has to be related to outside objects. And the idea

MAYA

of causation is inseparable from time and space. (II. 135-36.)

3. As no man can jump out of his own self, so no man can go beyond the limits that have been put upon him by the laws of time and space. Every attempt to solve the laws of causation, time and space, would be futile, because the very attempt would have to be made by taking for granted the existence of these three. What does the statement of the existence of the world mean, then? "This world has no existence." What is meant by that? It means that it has no absolute existence. It exists only in relation to my mind, to your mind, and to the mind of everyone else. We see this world with the five senses, but if we had another sense, we would see in it something more. If we had yet another sense, it would appear as something still different. It has, therefore, no real existence; it has no unchangeable, immovable, infinite existence. Nor can it be called non-existence, seeing that it exists, and we have to work in and through it. It is a mixture of existence and non-existence. (II. 91.)

4. What you call matter, or spirit, or mind, or anything else you may like to call them, the fact remains the same, we cannot say that they are, we cannot say that they are not. This eternal play of light and darkness, indiscriminate,

indistinguishable, inseparable, is always there. A fact, yet, at the same time, not a fact; awake, and at the same time, asleep. This is a statement of facts, and this is what is called Maya. We are born in this Maya, we live in it, we think in it, we dream in it. We are philosophers in it, we are spiritual men in it, nay, we are devils in this Maya, and we are gods in this Maya. Stretch your ideas as far as you can, make them higher and higher, call them infinite, or by any other name you please, even these ideas are within this Maya. It cannot be otherwise, and the whole of human knowledge is generalisation of this Maya, trying to know it as it appears to be. This is the work of Nama Rupa—name and form. Everything that has form, everything that calls up an idea in your mind is within Maya, for everything that is bound by the laws of time, space, and causation is within Maya. (II. 112.)

5. This theory of Maya has been the most difficult thing to understand in all ages. Let me tell you in a few words that it is surely no theory, it is the combination of the three ideas of Desha-kala-nimitta—space, time, and causation—and this time and space and cause have been further reduced into Nama Rupa. Suppose there is a wave in the ocean. The wave is distinct from the ocean only in its form and name, and this form and this name cannot have any separate

existence from the wave; they exist only with the wave. The wave may subside, but the same amount of water remains, even if the name and form that were on the wave vanish for ever. So this Maya is what makes the difference between me and you, between all animals and man, between gods and men. In fact, it is this Maya that causes the Atman to be caught, as it were, in so many millions of beings, and these are distinguishable only through name and form. If you leave it alone, let name and form go, all this variety vanishes for ever, and you are what you really are. This is Maya. (III. 419-20.)

6. According to the Advaitists proper, the followers of Shankaracharya, the whole universe is the *apparent* evolution of God. God is the material cause of this universe, but not really, only apparently. The celebrated illustration used is that of the rope and the snake, where the rope appeared to be the snake, but was not really so. The rope did not really change into the snake. Even so this whole universe as it exists, is that Being. It is unchanged, and all the changes we see in it are only apparent. These changes are caused by Desha, Kala, and Nimitta (space, time, and causation), or, according to a higher psychological generalisation, by Nama and Rupa (name and form). It is by name and form that one thing is differentiated from another. The name and

form alone cause the difference. In reality, they are one and the same. Again, it is not, the Vedantists say, that there is something as phenomenon and something as noumenon. The rope is changed into the snake apparently only; and when the delusion ceases, the snake vanishes. When one is in ignorance, he sees the phenomenon and does not see God. When he sees God, this universe vanishes entirely for him. Ignorance or Maya, as it is called, is the cause of all this phenomenon—the Absolute, the Unchangeable, being taken as this manifested universe. It is defined as neither existence nor non-existence. It is not existence, because that can be said only of the Absolute, the Unchangeable, and in this sense, Maya is non-existence. Again, it cannot be said it is non-existence; for if it were, it could never produce the phenomenon. So it is something which is neither; and in the Vedanta philosophy it is called Anirvachaniya or inexpressible. (I. 363-64.)

7. A legend tells how once Narada said to Krishna, "Lord, show me Maya". A few days passed away, and Krishna asked Narada to make a trip with him towards a desert, and after walking for several miles, Krishna said, "Narada, I am thirsty; can you fetch some water for me?" "I will go at once, sir, and get you water." So Narada went. At a little distance there was a

village; he entered the village in search of water, and knocked at a door, which was opened by a most beautiful young girl. At the sight of her he immediately forgot that his Master was waiting for water, perhaps dying for the want of it. He forgot everything, and began to talk with the girl. All that day he did not return to his Master. The next day, he was again at the house, talking to the girl. That talk ripened into love; he asked the father for the daughter, and they were married, and lived there and had children. Thus twelve years passed. His father-in-law died, he inherited his property. He lived, as he seemed to think, a very happy life with his wife and children, his fields and his cattle, and so forth. Then came a flood. One night the river rose until it overflowed its banks and flooded the whole village. Houses fell, men and animals were swept away and drowned, and everything was floating in the rush of the stream. Narada had to escape. With one hand he held his wife, and with the other two of his children; another child was on his shoulders, and he was trying to ford the tremendous flood. After a few steps he found the current was too strong, and the child on his shoulders fell and was borne away. A cry of despair came from Narada. In trying to save that child, he lost his grasp upon one of the others, and it also was lost. At last his wife, whom he clasped with all his might, was torn away by the current, and he was thrown on the bank, weeping and wailing in bitter lamentation. Behind him there came a gentle voice, "My child, where is the water? You went to fetch a pitcher of water, and I am waiting for you; you have gone for quite half an hour." "Half an hour!" Narada exclaimed. Twelve whole years had passed through his mind, and all these scenes had happened in half an hour! And this is Maya. (II. 120-21.)

XXXII

MEDITATION

1. The mind tries to think of one object, to hold itself to one particular spot, as the top of the head, the heart, etc., and if the mind succeeds in receiving the sensations only through that part of the body, and through no other part, that would be Dharana, and when the mind succeeds in keeping itself in that state for some time it is called Dhyana (meditation). (I. 270.)

2. That (meditation) is the highest state.... When (the mind) is doubtful that is not its great state. Its great state is meditation. It looks upon things and sees things, not identifying itself with anything else. As long as I feel pain, I have identified myself with the body. When I feel joy or pleasure, I have identified myself with the body. But the high state will look with the same pleasure or blissfulness upon pleasure or upon pain.... Every meditation is direct super-consciousness. In perfect concentration the soul becomes actually free from the bonds of the gross body and knows itself as it is. (IV. 226.)

3. Meditation is the focussing of the mind on some object. If the mind acquires concentration on one object, it can be so concentrated on any object whatsoever. (VI. 486.)

4. First, the practice of meditation has to

proceed with some one object before the mind. Once I used to concentrate my mind on some black point. Ultimately, during those days, I could not see the point any more, nor notice that the point was before me at all—the mind used to be no more—no wave of functioning would rise, as if it were all an ocean without any breath of air. In that state I used to experience glimpses of supersensuous truth. So I think, the practice of meditation even with some trifling external object leads to mental concentration. But it is true that the mind very easily attains calmness when one practises meditation with anything on which one's mind is most apt to settle down. This is the reason why we have in this country so much worship of the images of gods and goddesses. And what wonderful art developed from such worship! But no more of that now. The fact however is that the objects of meditation can never be the same in the case of all men. People have proclaimed and preached to others only those external objects to which they held on to become perfected in meditation. Oblivious of the fact, later on, that these objects are aids to the attainment of perfect mental calmness, men have extolled them beyond everything else. They have wholly concerned themselves with the means, getting comparatively unmindful of the end. The real aim is to make the mind functionless, but this cannot be got at unless one becomes absorbed in some object. (VI. 486-87.)

5. Within there is the lion—the eternally pure, illumined and ever-free Atman; and directly one realises Him through meditation and concentration, this world of Maya vanishes. (VII. 253.)

6. You must keep the mind fixed on one object, like an unbroken stream of oil. The ordinary man's mind is scattered on different objects, and at the time of meditation, too, the mind is at first apt to wander. But let any desire whatever arise in the mind, you must sit calmly and watch what sort of ideas are coming. By continuing to watch in that way, the mind becomes calm, and there are no thought-waves in it. These waves represent the thought-activity of the mind. Those things that you have previously thought too deeply, have transformed themselves into a subconscious current, and therefore these come up in the mind in meditation. The rise of these waves, or thoughts, during meditation is an evidence that your mind is tending towards concentration. Sometimes the mind is concentrated on a set of ideas—this is called meditation with Vikalpa or oscillation. But when the mind becomes almost free from all activities, it melts in the inner Self, which is the essence of infinite Knowledge, One and Itself Its own support. (VII. 253-54.)

7. The greatest help to spiritual life is

meditation. In meditation we divest ourselves of all material conditions and feel our divine nature. We do not depend upon any external help in meditation. (II. 37.)

8. The greatest thing is meditation. It is the nearest approach to spiritual life—the mind meditating. It is the one moment in our daily life that we are not material—the Soul thinking of Itself, free from all matter—this marvellous touch of the Soul. (V. 253.)

9. Think and meditate that you are the omnipresent Atman. "I am neither the body, nor the mind, nor the Buddhi (determining faculty), neither the gross nor the subtle body,"—by this process of elimination, immerse your mind in the transcendent knowledge which is your real nature. Kill the mind by thus plunging it repeatedly in this. Then only you will realise the Essence of Intelligence, or be established in your real nature. Knower and known, meditator and object meditated upon, will then become one, and the cessation of all phenomenal superimpositions will follow.... There is no relative or conditioned knowledge in this state. When the Atman is the only knower, by what means can you possibly know it? The Atman is knowledge, the Atman is Intelligence, the Atman is Sachchidananda. (VII. 196.)

10. Samadhi is the property of every human

being—nay, every animal. From the lowest animal to the highest angel, some time or other, each one will have to come to that state, and then, and then alone, will real religion begin for him. Until then we only struggle towards that stage. There is no difference now between us and those who have no religion, because we have no experience. What is concentration good for, save to bring us to this experience? Each one of the steps to attain Samadhi has been reasoned out, properly adjusted, scientifically organised, and, when faithfully practised, will surely lead us to the desired end. Then will all sorrows cease, all miseries vanish; the seeds for actions will be burnt, and the soul will be free for ever. (I. 188.)

XXXIII

MIND AND THOUGHT

1. The highest men are calm, silent and unknown. They are the men who really know the power of thought; they are sure that, even if they go into a cave and close the door and simply think five true thoughts and then pass away, these five thoughts of theirs will live through eternity. Indeed such thoughts will penetrate through the mountains, cross the oceans, and travel through the world. (I. 106.)

2. Take up one idea. Make that one idea your life; think of it; dream of it; live on that idea. Let the brain, muscles, nerves, every part of your body be full of that idea, and just leave every other idea alone. This is the way to success, and this is the way great spiritual giants are produced. (I. 177.)

3. All minds are the same, different parts of one Mind. He who knows one lump of clay has known all the clay in the universe. He who knows and controls his own mind, knows the secret of every mind, and has power over every mind. (II. 17.)

4. There have been omniscient men, and, I believe, there will be yet; and there will be myriads of them in the cycles to come. (I. 28.)

MIND AND THOUGHT

5. It is thought which is the propelling force in us. Fill the mind with the highest thoughts, hear them day after day, think them month after month. Never mind failures; they are quite natural, they are the beauty of life, these failures. (II. 152.)

6. When your mind has become controlled you have control over the whole body; instead of being a slave to this machine, the machine is your slave. Instead of this machine being able to drag the soul down it becomes its greatest helpmate. (I. 265.)

7. Mind is like a lake, and every thought is like a wave upon that lake. Just as in the lake waves rise, and then fall down and disappear, so these thought-waves are continually rising in the mind-stuff, and then disappearing, but they do not disappear for ever. They become finer and finer, but they are all there, ready to start up at another time, when called upon to do so. (II. 268-69.)

8. Just as unconscious work is beneath consciousness, so there is another work which is above consciousness, and which also is not accompanied with the feeling of egoism. The feeling of egoism is only on the middle plane. When the mind is above or below that line there is no feeling of "I", and yet the mind works. When the mind goes beyond this line of

self-consciousness it is called Samadhi or super-consciousness. (I. 180.)

9. When the mind is free from activity or functioning, it vanishes and the Self is revealed. This state has been described by the commentator Shankara as अपरोक्षानुभूतिः or supersensuous state. (VI. 475.)

10. Each thought is a little hammer blow on the lump of iron which our bodies are, manufacturing out of it what we want to be. (VII. 20.)

11. We are what our thoughts have made us; so take care of what you think. (VII. 14.)

12. Every vicious thought will rebound, every thought of hatred which you have thought, in a cave even, is stored up, and will one day come back to you with tremendous power in the form of some misery here. If you project hatred and jealousy, they will rebound on you with compound interest. No power can avert them; when once you have put them in motion you will have to bear them. Remembering this will prevent you from doing wicked things. (I. 262.)

13. We are heirs to all the good thoughts of the universe, if we open ourselves to them. (VII. 20.)

14. My idea is to bring to the door of the meanest, the poorest, the noble ideas that the human race has developed both in and out of India, and let them think for themselves....

MIND AND THOUGHT

Liberty of thought and action is the only condition of life, of growth and well-being. Where it does not exist, the man, the race, the nation must go down.... Caste or no caste, creed or no creed, any man, or class, or caste, or nation, or institution which bars the power of free thought and action of an individual—even so long as that power does not injure others—is devilish and must go down. (V. 28-29.)

XXXIV

MOHAMMED AND ISLAM

1. Mohammed—the Messenger of equality. You ask, "What good can there be in his religion?" If there was no good, how could it live? The good alone lives, that alone survives.... How could Mohammedanism have lived, had there been nothing good in its teaching? There is much good. (IV. 133.)

2. Mohammed was the Prophet of equality, of the brotherhood of man, the brotherhood of all Mussulmans. (IV. 133.)

3. Mohammed by his life showed that amongst the Mohammedans there should be perfect equality and brotherhood. There was no question of race, caste, colour or sex. The Sultan of Turkey may buy a Negro from the mart of Africa, and bring him in chains to Turkey; but should he become a Mohammedan, and have sufficient merit and abilities, he might even marry the daughter of the Sultan. Compare this with the way in which the Negroes and the American Indians are treated in this country! And what do Hindus do? If one of your missionaries chance to touch the food of an orthodox person, he would throw it away. Notwithstanding our grand philosophy you note our weakness in practice;

MOHAMMED AND ISLAM

but there you see the greatness of the Mohammedan beyond other races, showing itself in equality, perfect equality regardless of race or colour. (IV. 133-34.)

4. The fact that all these old religions are living today, proves that they must have kept that mission intact; in spite of all their mistakes, in spite of all difficulties, in spite of all quarrels, in spite of all the incrustation of forms and figures, the heart of everyone of them is sound —it is a throbbing, beating, living heart. They have not lost, any one of them, the great mission they came for. And it is splendid to study that mission. Take Mohammedanism, for instance.... As soon as a man becomes a Mohammedan, the whole of Islam receives him as a brother with open arms, without making any distinction, which no other religion does. If one of your American Indians becomes a Mohammedan, the Sultan of Turkey would have no objection to dine with him. If he has brains, no position is barred to him. In this country, I have never yet seen a church where the white man and the Negro can kneel side by side to pray. (II. 371.)

5. Islam makes its followers all equal—so, that is the peculiar excellence of Mohammedanism. ... What Mohammedanism comes to preach to the world in this practical brotherhood of all belonging to their faith. (II. 371.)

6. Among Mohammedans the Prophets and great and noble persons are worshipped, and they turn their faces towards the Caaba when they pray. These things show that men at the first stage of religious development have to make use of something external, and when the inner self becomes purified they turn to more abstract perceptions. (III. 362.)

7. It is a mistaken statement that has been made to us that the Mohammedans do not believe that women have souls. I am very sorry to say it is an old mistake among Christian people, and they seem to like the mistake.... By the by, you know I am not a Mohammedan, but yet I have had opportunities for studying them, and there is not one word in the Koran which says that women have no souls, but in fact it says they have. (IV. 192.)

8. England has the sword, the material world, as our Mohammedan conquerors had before her. Yet Akbar the Great became practically a Hindu; educated Mohammedans, the Sufis, are hardly to be distinguished from the Hindus; they do not eat beef, and in other ways conform to our usages. Their thought has become permeated by ours. (V. 195.)

9. Vedantic spirit of religious liberality has very much affected Mohammedanism. Mohammedanism in India is quite a different thing from

that in any other country. It is only when Mohammedans come from other countries and preach to their co-religionists in India about living with men who are not of their faith that a Mohammedan mob is aroused, and fights. (V. 310.)

10. Whether we call it Vedantism or any *ism*, the truth is that Advaitism is the last word of religion and thought and the only position from which one can look upon all religions and sects with love. We believe it is the religion of the future enlightened humanity. The Hindus may get the credit of arriving at it earlier than other races, they being an older race than either the Hebrew or the Arab; yet practical Advaitism, which looks upon and behaves to all mankind as one's own soul, is yet to be developed among the Hindus universally.

On the other hand, our experience is that if ever the followers of any religion approached to this equality in an appreciable degree in the plane of practical workaday life—it may be quite unconscious generally of the deeper meaning and the underlying principle of such conduct, which the Hindus, as a rule, so clearly perceive—it is those of Islam and Islam alone. (VI. 415.)

11. Therefore we are firmly persuaded that without the help of practical Islam, theories of Vedantism, however fine and wonderful they

may be, are entirely valueless to the vast mass of mankind. (VI. 415-16.)

12. For our own motherland a junction of the two great systems, Hinduism and Islam—Vedanta brain and Islam body—is the only hope. (VI. 416.)

13. I see in my mind's eye the future perfect India rising out of this chaos and strife, glorious and invincible, with Vedanta brain and Islam body. (VI. 416.)

XXXV

NON-INJURY

1. Never producing pain by thought, word and deed, in any living being, is what is called Ahimsa, non-injury. There is no virtue higher than non-injury. There is no happiness higher than what a man obtains by this attitude of non-offensiveness to all creation. (I. 189.)

2. The test of Ahimsa is absence of jealousy. Any man may do a good deed or make a good gift on the spur of the moment, or under the pressure of some superstition or priestcraft; but the real lover of mankind is he who is jealous of none. The so-called great men of the world may all be seen to become jealous of each other for a small name, for a little fame, and for a few bits of gold. So long as this jealousy exists in a heart, it is far away from the perfection of Ahimsa. The cow does not eat meat, nor does the sheep. Are they great Yogis, great non-injurers (Ahimsakas)? Any fool may abstain from eating this or that; surely that gives him no more distinction than to herbivorous animals. The man who will mercilessly cheat widows and orphans, and do the vilest deeds for money, is worse than any brute, even if he lives entirely on grass alone. The man whose heart never

cherishes even the thought of injury to any one, who rejoices at the prosperity of even his greatest enemy, that man is the Bhakta, he is the Yogi, he is the Guru of all, even though he lives every day of his life on the flesh of swine. Therefore we must always remember that external practices have value only as helps to develop internal purity. It is better to have internal purity alone, when minute attention to external observances is not practicable. But woe unto the man and woe unto the nation, that forgets the real, internal, spiritual essentials of religion, and mechanically clutches with death-like grasp at all external forms and never lets them go. (III. 67-68.)

3. Non-injuring has to be attained by him who would be free. No one is more powerful than he who has attained perfect non-injuring. No one could fight, no one could quarrel, in his presence. Yes, his very presence, and nothing else, means peace, means love wherever he may be. Nobody could be angry or fight in his presence. Even the animals, ferocious animals, would be peaceful before him. (VI. 126.)

4. All great teachers have taught, "Resist not evil", that non-resistance is the highest moral ideal. We all know that, if a certain number of us attempted to put that maxim fully into practice, the whole social fabric would fall to pieces, the wicked would take possession of our

properties and our lives, and would do whatever they liked with us. Even if only one day of such non-resistance were practised it would lead to disaster. Yet, intuitively, in our heart of hearts we feel the truth of the teaching "Resist not evil". This seems to us to be the highest ideal; yet to teach this doctrine only would be equivalent to condemning a vast portion of mankind. Not only so, it would be making men feel that they were always doing wrong, and cause in them scruples of conscience in all their actions; it would weaken them, and that constant self-disapproval would breed more vice than any other weakness would. (I. 37.)

5. Inactivity should be avoided by all means. Activity always means resistance. Resist all evils, mental and physical; and when you have succeeded in resisting, then will calmness come. It is very easy to say, "Hate nobody, resist not evil", but we know what that kind generally means in practice. When the eyes of society are turned towards us we may make a show of non-resistance, but in our hearts it is canker all the time.... This is hypocrisy and will serve no purpose. (I. 40.)

6. "To his enemies the householder must be a hero. Then he must resist. That is the duty of the householder. He must not sit down in a corner and weep, and talk nonsense about non-

resistance. If he does not show himself a hero to his enemies, he has not done his duty." (I. 44.)

7. This is a great lesson for us all to learn, that in all matters the two extremes are alike; the extreme positive and the extreme negative are always similar; when the vibrations of light are too slow we do not see them, nor do we see them when they are too rapid. So with sound; when very low in pitch we do not hear it, when very high we do not hear it either. Of like nature is the difference between resistance and non-resistance. One man does not resist because he is weak, lazy, and cannot, not because he will not; the other man knows that he can strike an irresistible blow if he likes; yet he not only does not strike, but blesses his enemies. The one who from weakness resists not commits a sin, and as such cannot receive any benefit from the non-resistance; while the other would commit a sin by offering resistance. (I. 38.)

XXXVI

ONENESS

1. The Omnipresent, the One without a second, the one without a body, the one great poet of the universe whose metre is the sun and stars, is giving to each what he deserves. (VI. 87.)

2. In this world of many, he who sees the One, in this ever-changing world, he who sees Him who never changes, as the Soul of his own soul, as his own Self, he is free, he is blessed, he has reached the goal. (II. 236.)

3. He who sees in this world of manifoldness that One running through all, in this world of death, he who finds that One Infinite Life, and in this world of insentience and ignorance, he who finds that One Light and Knowledge, unto him belongs eternal peace. Unto none else, unto none else. (II. 117.)

4. He is the One, the Creator of all, the Ruler of all, the Internal Soul of every being, He who makes His Oneness manifold. Thus sages who realise Him as the Soul of their souls, unto them belongs eternal peace; unto none else, unto none else. (II. 183.)

5. This is a good point to understand—that the sum and substance of this lecture is that there is but One Existence and that One Exist-

ence seen through different constitutions appears either as the earth, or heaven, or hell, or gods, or ghosts, or men, or demons, or world, or all these things. But among these many, "He who sees that One in this ocean of death, he who sees that One Life in this floating universe, who realises that One who never changes, unto him belongs eternal peace; unto none else, unto none else." (III. 24.)

6. One atom in this universe cannot move without dragging the whole world along with it. There cannot be any progress without the whole world following in the wake, and it is becoming every day clearer that the solution of any problem can never be attained on racial, or national, or narrow grounds. (III. 269.)

7. The God in you is the God in all. If you have not known this, you have known nothing. How can there be difference? It is all one. Every being is the temple of the Most High; if you can see that, good, if not, spirituality has yet to come to you. (I. 429.)

8. What good is it if we acknowledge in our prayers that God is the Father of us all, and in our daily lives do not treat every man as brother? (IV. 191.)

9. Every human personality may be compared to a glass globe. There is the same pure white light—an emission of the divine Being—in the

ONENESS

centre of each, but the glass being of different colours and thickness, the rays assume diverse aspects in the transmission. (IV. 191.)

10. Each is responsible for the evil anywhere in the world.... All that unites with the universal is virtue. All that separates is sin. You are a part of the Infinite. This is your nature. Hence you are your brother's keeper.... Not one can attain liberty until every being (ant or dog) has liberty. Not one can be happy until all are happy. When you hurt anyone you hurt yourself, for you and your brother are one. (VI. 83.)

11. Expansion is life, contraction is death. Love is life and hatred is death. (IV. 366.)

12. I am thoroughly convinced that no individual or nation can live by holding itself apart from the community of others, and whenever such an attempt has been made under false ideas of greatness, policy or holiness—the result has always been disastrous to the secluding one. (IV. 365.)

XXXVII

RAMAKRISHNA

1. The time was ripe for one to be born, the embodiment of both this head and heart; the time was ripe for one to be born, who in one body would have the brilliant intellect of Shankara and the wonderfully expansive, infinite heart of Chaitanya; one who would see in every sect the same spirit working, the same God; one who would see God in every being, one whose heart would weep for the poor, for the weak, for the outcast, for the downtrodden, for every one in this world, inside India or outside India; and at the same time whose grand brilliant intellect would conceive of such noble thoughts as would harmonise all conflicting sects, not only in India but outside of India, and bring a marvellous harmony, the universal religion of head and heart into existence. Such a man was born, and I had the good fortune to sit at his feet for years. The time was ripe, it was necessary that such a man should be born, and he came; and the most wonderful part of it was, that his life's work was just near a city which was full of Western thought, a city which had run mad after these occidental ideas, a city which had become more Europeanised than any other city in India. There

he lived, without any book-learning whatsoever; this great intellect never learnt even to write his own name, but the most brilliant graduates of our university found in him an intellectual giant. He was a strange man, this Shri Ramakrishna Paramahamsa. It is a long, long story, and I have no time to tell anything about him tonight. Let me now only mention the great Shri Ramakrishna, the fulfilment of the Indian sages, the sage for the time, one whose teaching is just now, in the present time, most beneficial. And mark the divine power working behind the man. The son of a poor priest, born in an out-of-the-way village, unknown and unthought of, today is worshipped literally by thousands in Europe and America, and tomorrow will be worshipped by thousands more. (III. 267-68.)

2. Now, all the ideas that I preach are only an attempt to echo his ideas. Nothing is mine originally except the wicked ones, everything I say which is false and wicked. But every word that I have ever uttered which is true and good, is simply an attempt to echo his voice. (VIII. 79.)

3. Our heroes must be spiritual. Such a hero has been given to us in the person of Ramakrishna Paramahamsa. If this nation wants to rise, take my word for it, it will have to rally enthusiastically round this name. It does not matter who preaches Ramakrishna Paramahamsa,

whether I, or you, or anybody else. But him I place before you, and it is for you to judge, and for the good of our race, for the good of our nation, to judge now, what you shall do with this great ideal of life. One thing we are to remember, that it was the purest of all lives that you have ever seen, or let me tell you distinctly, that you have ever read of. And before you is the fact that it is the most marvellous manifestation of soul-power that you can read of, much less expect to see. Within ten years of his passing away, this power has encircled the globe; that fact is before you. In duty bound, therefore, for the good of our race, for the good of our religion, I place this great spiritual ideal before you. Judge him not through me. I am only a weak instrument. Let not his character be judged by seeing me. It was so great that if I or any other of his disciples spent hundreds of lives, we could not do justice to a millionth part of what he really was. Judge for yourselves; in the heart of your hearts is the Eternal Witness, and may He, the same Ramakrishna Paramahamsa, for the good of our nation, for the welfare of our country, and for the good of humanity, open your hearts, make you true and steady to work for the immense change which must come, whether we exert ourselves or not. For, the work of the Lord does not wait for the like of you or me. He can raise His workers from the dust by hundreds and by thousands. It is a glory and a privilege that we are allowed to work at all under Him. (III. 315-16.)

4. If there has been anything achieved by me, by thoughts, or words, or deeds, if from my lips has ever fallen one word that has helped any one in the world, I lay no claim to it, it was his. But if there have been curses falling from my lips, if there has been hatred coming out of me, it is all mine, and not his. All that has been weak has been mine, and all that has been life-giving, strengthening, pure, and holy, has been his inspiration, his words, and he himself. Yes, my friends, the world has yet to know that man. We read in the history of the world about prophets and their lives, and these come down to us through centuries of writings and workings by their disciples. Through thousands of years of chiselling and modelling, the lives of the great prophets of yore come down to us; and yet, in my opinion, not one stands so high in brilliance as that life which I saw with my own eyes, under whose shadow I have lived, at whose feet I have learnt everything—the life of Ramakrishna Paramahamsa. (III. 312-13.)

5. He had found that the one idea in all religions is, "not me, but Thou", and he who says, "not me", the Lord fills his heart. The less of

this little "I" the more of God there is in him. That he found to be the truth in every religion in the world, and he set himself to accomplish this.... Whenever he wanted to do anything he never confined himself to fine theories, but would enter into the practice immediately. We see many persons talking the most wonderfully fine things about charity and about equality and the rights of other people and all that, but it is only in theory. I was so fortunate as to find one who was able to carry theory into practice. (IV. 174.)

6. Our teacher would never touch a coin with his hands. He took just the little food offered, just so many yards of cotton cloth, no more. He could never be induced to take any other gift. (VIII. 80.)

7. In the presence of my Master I found out that man could be perfect, even in this body. Those lips never cursed any one, never even criticised any one. Those eyes were beyond the possibility of seeing evil, that mind had lost the power of thinking evil. He saw nothing but good. That tremendous purity, that tremendous renunciation is the one secret of spirituality. (IV. 183.)

8. He was a triumphant example, a living realisation of the complete conquest of lust and of desire for money. He was beyond all ideas of either, and such men are necessary for this

century. Such renunciation is necessary in these days when men have begun to think that they cannot live a month without what they call their "necessities", and which they are increasing out of all proportion. It is necessary in a time like this that a man should arise to demonstrate to the sceptics of the world that there yet breathes a man who does not care a straw for all the gold or all the fame that is in the universe. (IV. 184.)

9. He always said, "If any good comes from my lips, it is the Mother who speaks; what have I to do with it?" That was his one idea about his work, and to the day of his death he never gave it up. This man sought no one. His principle was, first form character, first earn spirituality and results will come of themselves. His favourite illustration was, "When the lotus opens, the bees come of their own accord to seek the honey; so let the lotus of your character be full-blown, and the results will follow." This is a great lesson to learn. (IV. 177.)

10. Spirituality can be communicated just as really as I can give you a flower. This is true in the most literal sense.... Know Truth for yourself, and there will be many to whom you can teach it afterwards; they will all come. This was the attitude of my Master. (IV. 178.)

11. People came by thousands to see and hear this wonderful man, who spoke in a *patois*, every

word of which was forceful and instinct with light. For it is not what is spoken, much less the language in which it is spoken, but it is the personality of the speaker which dwells in everything he says that carries weight.... The words of a man who can put his personality into them, take effect, but he must have tremendous personality. (IV. 178.)

12. I have read about Buddha and Christ and Mohammed, about all those different luminaries of ancient times, how they would stand up and say, "Be thou whole," and the man became whole. I now found it to be true, and when I myself saw this man, all scepticism was brushed aside. It could be done, and my Master used to say, "Religion can be given and taken more tangibly, more really than anything else in the world." Be therefore spiritual first; have something to give, and then stand before the world and give it. (IV. 179.)

13. From actual experience, he came to know that the goal of every religion is the same, that each is trying to teach the same thing, the difference being largely in method and still more in language. At the core, all sects and all religions have the same aim. (IV. 174.)

14. My Master's message to mankind is: "Be spiritual and realise truth for yourself." He would have you give up for the sake of your fellow-

beings. He would have you cease talking about love for your brother, and set to work to prove your words. The time has come for renunciation, for realisation; and then you will see the harmony in all the religions of the world. You will know that there is no need of any quarrel. And then only will you be ready to help humanity. To proclaim and make clear the fundamental unity underlying all religions was the mission of my Master. Other teachers have taught special religions which bear their names, but this great teacher of the nineteenth century made no claim for himself. He left every religion undisturbed because he had realised that, in reality, they are all part and parcel of the one eternal religion. (IV. 187.)

15. Bhagavân Sri Ramakrishna incarnated himself in India, to demonstrate what the true religion of the Aryan race is; to show where amidst all its many divisions and offshoots, scattered over the land in the course of its immemorial history, lies the true unity of the Hindu religion, which by its overwhelming number of sects discordant to superficial view, quarrelling constantly with each other and abounding in customs divergent in every way, has constituted itself a misleading enigma for our countrymen and the butt of contempt for foreigners; and, above all, to hold up before

men, for their lasting welfare, as a living embodiment of the Sanatana Dharma, his own wonderful life into which he infused the universal spirit and character of this Dharma, so long cast into oblivion by the process of time. (VI. 183-84.)

16. The life of Sri Ramakrishna was an extraordinary searchlight under whose illumination one is able to really understand the whole scope of Hindu religion. He was the object-lesson of all the theoretical knowledge given in the Shâstras. He showed by his life what the Rishis and Avatâras really wanted to teach. The books were theories, he was the realisation. This man had in fifty-one years lived the five thousand years of national spiritual life, and so raised himself to be an object-lesson for future generations. The Vedas can only be explained and the Shastras reconciled by his theory of Avasthâ or stages —that we must not only tolerate others, but positively embrace them, and that truth is the basis of all religions. (V. 53.)

17. At the very dawn of this momentous epoch, the reconciliation of all aspects and ideals of religious thought and worship is being proclaimed; this boundless, all-embracing idea had been lying inherent, but so long concealed, in the Religion Eternal and its scriptures, and now

rediscovered, it is being declared to humanity in a trumpet voice.

This epochal new dispensation is the harbinger of great good to the whole world, specially to India; and the inspirer of this dispensation, Sri Bhagavan Ramakrishna, is the reformed and remodelled manifestation of all the past great epoch-makers in religion. O man, have faith in this, and lay it to heart.

The dead never return; the past night does not reappear; a spent-up tidal wave does not rise anew: neither does man inhabit the same body over again. So from the worship of the dead past, O man, we invite you to the worship of the living present; from the regretful brooding over bygones, we invite you to the activities of the present; from the waste of energy in retracing lost and demolished pathways, we call you back to broad new-laid highways lying very near. He that is wise, let him understand.

Of that power which at the very first impulse has roused distant echoes from all the four quarters of the globe, conceive in your mind the manifestation in its fulness; and discarding all idle misgivings, weaknesses and the jealousies characteristic of enslaved peoples, come and help in the turning of this mighty wheel of new dispensation!

With the conviction firmly rooted in your heart

that you are the servants of the Lord, His children, helpers in the fulfilment of His purposes, enter the arena of work. (VI. 185-86.)

XXXVIII

RELIGION

1. Religion is the manifestation of the Divinity already in man. (IV. 358.)

2. As so many rivers, having their source in different mountains, roll down, crooked or straight, and at last come into the ocean—so, all these various creeds and religions, taking their start from different standpoints and running through crooked or straight courses, at last come unto Thee. (I. 390.)

3. The proof of one religion depends on the proof of all the rest. For instance, if I have six fingers, and no one else has, you may well say that is abnormal. The same reasoning may be applied to the argument that only one religion is true and all others false. One religion only, like one set of six fingers in the world, would be unnatural. We see, therefore, that if one religion is true, all others must be true. There are differences in non-essentials, but in essentials they are all one. If my five fingers are true, they prove that your five fingers are true too. (I. 318.)

4. Is religion to justify itself by the discoveries of reason, through which every other concrete science justifies itself? Are the same methods of investigation which we apply to sciences and

knowledge outside, to be applied to the science of Religion? In my opinion, this must be so, and I am also of opinion that the sooner it is done the better. If a religion is destroyed by such investigations, it was then all the time useless, unworthy superstition; and the sooner it goes the better. I am thoroughly convinced that its destruction would be the best thing that could happen. All that is dross will be taken off, no doubt, but the essential parts of religion will emerge triumphant out of this investigation. Not only will it be made scientific, as scientific, at least, as any of the conclusions of physics or chemistry, but will have greater strength, because physics or chemistry has no internal mandate to vouch for its truth, which religion has. (I. 367.)

5. Religion must be studied on a broader basis than formerly. All narrow, limited, fighting ideas of religion have to go. All sect ideas and tribal or national ideas of religion must be given up. That each tribe or nation should have its own particular God, and think that every other is wrong, is a superstition that should belong to the past. All such ideas must be abandoned. (II. 67.)

6. Now comes the question, can religion really accomplish anything? It can. It brings to man eternal life. It has made man what he is and will

make of this human animal a God. That is what religion can do. Take religion from human society and what will remain? Nothing but a forest of brutes. Sense-happiness is not the goal of humanity. Wisdom (Jnana) is the goal of all life. We find that man enjoys his intellect more than an animal enjoys its senses, and we see that man enjoys his spiritual nature even more than his rational nature. So the highest wisdom must be this spiritual knowledge. With this knowledge will come bliss. All these things of this world are but the shadows, the manifestations in the third or fourth degree of the real Knowledge and Bliss. (III. 4.)

7. The chief thing is to *want* God. We want everything except God, because our ordinary wants are supplied by the external world; it is only when our necessities have gone beyond the external world that we want a supply from the internal, from God. So long as our needs are confined within the narrow limits of this physical universe, we cannot have any need for God, it is only when we have become satiated with everything here, that we look beyond for a supply. It is only when the need is there that the demand will come. Have done with this child's play of the world as soon as you can, and then you will feel the necessity of something beyond the

world, and the first step in religion will come. (IV. 19.)

8. As my Master used to say, what would you think of men who went into a mango orchard, and busied themselves in counting the leaves, and examining the colour of the leaves, the size of the twigs, the number of branches, and so forth, while only one of them had the sense to begin to eat the mangoes? So leave this counting of leaves and twigs, and this note-taking to others. That work has its own value in its proper place, but not here, in the spiritual realm. Men never become spiritual through such work; you have never once seen a strong spiritual man among these "leaf-counters". Religion is the highest aim of man, the highest glory, but it does not require "leaf-counting". If you want to be a Christian, it is not necessary to know whether Christ was born in Jerusalem or Bethlehem or just the exact date on which He pronounced the Sermon on the Mount; you only require to *feel* the Sermon on the Mount. It is not necessary to read two thousand words on when it was delivered. All this is for the enjoyment of the learned. Let them have it; say amen to that. Let *us* eat the mangoes. (IV. 25-26.)

9. Religion is its own end. That religion which is only a means to worldly well-being is not religion, whatever else it may be. (IV. 279.)

RELIGION

10. The end and aim of all religion is to realise God. The greatest of all training is to worship God alone. (VI. 82.)

11. Religion is one, but its application must be various. (VI. 82.)

12. No man is born to any religion; he has a religion in his own soul. (VI. 82.)

13. Religious quarrels are always over the husks. When purity, when spirituality goes, leaving the soul dry, quarrels begin, and not before. (VI. 127.)

14. Religion is the realising of God. (V. 417.)

15. True religion is entirely transcendental. Every being that is in the universe has the potentiality of transcending the senses; even the little worm will one day transcend the senses and reach God. No life will be a failure; there is no such thing as failure in the universe. (I. 416.)

16. With most people religion is a sort of intellectual assent and goes no further than a document. I would not call it religion. It is better to be an atheist than to have that sort of religion. (IV. 34.)

17. You must bear in mind that religion does not consist in talk, or doctrines or books, but in realisation; it is not learning but *being*. (IV. 35.)

18. We are all of us babies here; we may be old and have studied all the books in the universe, but we are all spiritual babies. We have

learnt the doctrines and dogmas, but realised nothing in our lives. (IV. 36.)

19. Man has an idea that there can be only one religion, that there can be only one Prophet, and that there can be only one Incarnation, but that idea is not true. By studying the lives of all these great messengers, we find that each, as it were, was destined to play a part, and a part only; that the harmony consists in the sum total, and not in one note. (IV. 120-21.)

20. Now in my little experience I have collected this knowledge: that in spite of all the devilry that religion is blamed with, religion is not at all in fault; no religion ever persecuted men, no religion ever burnt witches, no religion ever did any of these things. What then incited people to do these things? Politics, but never religion; and if such politics takes the name of religion whose fault is that? (IV. 125.)

21. There never was my religion or yours, my national religion or your national religion; there never existed many religions, there is only the one. One Infinite Religion existed all through eternity and will ever exist, and this Religion is expressing itself in various countries, in various ways. (IV. 180.)

21. I do not understand how people declare themselves to be believers in God, and at the same time think that God has handed over to a

little body of men all truth, and they are the guardians of the rest of humanity. (IV. 182.)

23. The whole world of religions is only a travelling, a coming up, of different men and women, through various conditions and circumstances, to the same goal. Every religion is only evolving a God out of the material man, and the same God is the inspirer of all of them. (I. 18.)

24. Man is to become divine by realising the divine; idols or temples or churches or books are only the supports, the helps, of his spiritual childhood: but on and on he must progress. (I. 16.)

25. Man must realise God, feel God, see God. talk of God. That is religion. (IV. 165.)

26. Love and charity for the whole human race, that is the test of true religiousness. (I. 325.)

27. Religion begins with a tremendous dissatisfaction with the present state of things, with our lives, and a hatred, an intense hatred, for this patching of life, an unbounded disgust for fraud and lies. (II. 123-24.)

28. "Death is better than a vegetating ignorant life; it is better to die on the battle-field than to live a life of defeat." This is the basis of religion. When a man takes this stand he is on the way to find the truth, he is on the way to God. (II. 124.)

29. That determination must be the first

impulse towards becoming religious. I will hew out a way for myself. I will know the truth, or give up my life in the attempt. For on this side it is nothing, it is gone, it is vanishing every day . . . on the other, there are the great charms of conquest, victories over all the ills of life, victory over life itself, the conquest of the universe. On that side men can stand. (II. 124.)

30. My Master used to say, the vulture rises higher and higher until he becomes a speck, but his eye is always on the piece of rotten carrion on the earth. After all, what is the result of your ideas of religion? To cleanse the streets and have more bread and clothes? Who cares for bread and clothes? Millions come and go every minute. Who cares? Why care for the joys and vicissitudes of this little world? Go beyond that if you dare; go beyond law, let the universe vanish, and stand alone. "I am Existence-Absolute, Knowledge-Absolute, Bliss-Absolute; I am He, I am He." (III. 18.)

31. Religion is realisation; not talk, nor doctrine, nor theories, however beautiful they may be. It is being and becoming, not hearing or acknowledging; it is the whole soul becoming changed into what it believes. (II. 396.)

32. Renunciation is the true background of all religious thoughts wherever it be, and you will always find that as this idea of renunciation

lessens, the more will the senses creep into the field of religion, and spirituality will decrease in the same ratio. (IV. 183-84.)

33. To put the Hindu ideas into English and then make out of dry philosophy and intricate mythology and queer startling psychology, a religion which shall be easy, simple, popular, and at the same time meet the requirements of the highest minds—is a task only those can understand who have attempted it. The abstract Advaita must become living—poetic—in everyday life; out of hopelessly intricate mythology must come concrete moral forms; and out of bewildering Yogi-ism must come the most scientific and practical psychology—and all this must be put in a form so that a child may grasp it. That is my life's work. (V. 104-05.)

34. What I want to propagate is a religion that will be equally acceptable to all minds; it must be equally philosophic, equally emotional, equally mystic, and equally conducive to action. If professors from the colleges come, scientific men and physicists, they will court reason. Let them have it as much as they want. . . . Similarly, if the mystic comes, we must welcome him, be ready to give him the science of mental analysis, and practically demonstrate it before him. And if emotional people come, we must sit, laugh, and weep with them in the name of

the Lord; we must "drink the cup of love and become mad". If the energetic worker comes, we must work with him, with all the energy that we have. And this combination will be the ideal of the nearest approach to a universal religion. Would to God that all men were so constituted that in their minds *all* these elements of philosophy, mysticism, emotion, and of work were equally present in full! That is the ideal, my ideal of a perfect man. Everyone who has only one or two of these elements of character, I consider "one-sided"; and this world is almost full of such "one-sided" men, with knowledge of that one road only in which they move; and anything else is dangerous and horrible to them. To become harmoniously balanced in all these four directions is *my* ideal of religion. (II. 387-88.)

35. If there is ever to be a universal religion, it must be one which will have no location in place or time, which will be infinite like the God it will preach, . . . which in its catholicity will embrace in its infinite arms, and find a place for every human being from the lowest grovelling savage not far removed from the brute to the highest man towering by the virtues of his head and heart almost above humanity, making society stand in awe of him and doubt his human nature, . . . which will have no place for persecu-

tion or intolerance in its polity, which will recognise divinity in every man and woman, and whose whole scope, whose whole force will be centred in aiding humanity to realise its own true, divine nature. (I. 19.)

XXXIX

SANNYASA OR THE MONASTIC LIFE

1. When a man has fulfilled the duties and obligations of that stage of life in which he is born, and his aspirations lead him to seek a spiritual life and to abandon altogether the worldly pursuits of possession, fame or power, when, by the growth of insight into the nature of the world, he sees its impermanence, its strife, its misery, and the paltry nature of its prizes, and turns away from all these—then he seeks the true, the Eternal Love, the Refuge. He makes complete renunciation (Sannyasa) of all worldly position, property and name, and wanders forth into the world to live a life of self-sacrifice and to persistently seek spiritual knowledge, striving to excêl in love and compassion and to acquire lasting insight. Gaining these pearls of wisdom by years of meditation, discipline and inquiry, he in his turn becomes a teacher and hands on to disciples, lay or professed, who may seek them from him, all that he can of wisdom and beneficence. (V. 260.)

2. A Sannyasin cannot belong to any religion, for his is a life of independent thought, which draws from all religions; his is a life of realisa-

SANNYASA OR THE MONASTIC LIFE

tion, not merely of theory or belief, much less of dogma. (V. 260.)

3. The real aim of Sannyasa is—आत्मनो मोक्षार्थं जगद्धिताय च—"For the highest freedom of the self and the good of the world." Without having Sannyasa none can really be a knower of Brahman—this is what the Vedas and the Vedanta proclaim. Don't listen to the words of those who say, "We shall both live the worldly life and be knowers of Brahman." That is the flattering self-consolation of crypto-pleasure-seekers. (VI. 504.)

4. No Freedom without renunciation. Highest love for God can never be achieved without renunciation. (VI. 505.)

5. Nobody attains Freedom without shaking off the coils of worldly worries. The very fact that somebody lives the worldly life proves that he is tied down to it as the bondslave of some craving or other. Why otherwise will he cling to that life at all? He is the slave either of lust or of gold, of position or of fame, of learning or of scholarship. It is only after freeing oneself from all this thraldom that one can get on along the way of Freedom. Let people argue as loud as they please, I have got this conviction that unless all these bonds are given up, unless the monastic life is embraced, none is going to be

saved, no attainment of Brahmajnana is possible. (VI. 505.)

6. For the good of the many, for the happiness of the many, is the Sannyasin born. His life is all vain, indeed, who, embracing Sannyasa, forgets this ideal. The Sannyasin, verily, is born into this world to lay down his life for others, to stop the bitter cries of men, to wipe the tears of the widow, to bring peace to the soul of the bereaved mother, to equip the ignorant masses for the struggle for existence, to accomplish the secular and spiritual well-being of all through the diffusion of spiritual teachings and to arouse the sleeping lion of Brahman in all by throwing in the light of knowledge. (VI. 511-12.)

7. Arise, awake; wake up yourself, and awaken others. Achieve the consummation of life before you pass off—"Arise, awake, and stop not till the goal is reached!" (VI. 512.)

8. Getting the human birth, when the desire for Freedom becomes very strong, and along with it comes the grace of a person of realisation, then men's desire for Self-knowledge becomes intensified. Otherwise the mind of men given to lust and wealth never inclines that way. How should the desire to know Brahman arise in one who has the hankering in his mind for the pleasure of family-life, for wealth and for fame? He who is prepared to renounce all, who amid

the strong current of the duality of good and evil, happiness and misery, is calm, steady, balanced, and awake to his Ideal, alone endeavours to attain to Self-knowledge. He alone by the might of his own power tears asunder the net of the world, निर्गच्छति जगज्जालात् पिञ्जरादिव केशरी।—one emerges like a lion, breaking the barriers of Maya. (VII. 193.)

9. One must have both internal and external Sannyasa—renunciation in spirit as well as formal renunciation.... Without dispassion for the world, without renunciation, without giving up the desire for enjoyment, absolutely nothing can be accomplished in the spiritual life. "It is not like a sweetmeat in the hands of a child which you can snatch by a trick." (VII. 193.)

10. There have been and are Sannyasins or monks in every known religion. There are Hindu monks, Buddhist monks, Christian monks, and even Islam had to yield its rigorous denial and take in whole orders of mendicant monks. (IV. 303.)

11. But then, what about this marvellous experience of standing alone, discarding all help, breasting the storms of life, of working without any sense of recompense, without any sense of putrid duty? Working a whole life, joyful, free—because not goaded on to work like slaves —by false human love or ambition?

This the monk alone can have. What about religion? Has it to remain or vanish? If it remains it requires its experts, its soldiers. The monk is the religious expert, having made religion his one *métier* of life. He is the soldier of God. What religion dies so long as it has a band of devoted monks? (IV. 307.)

12. Wheresoever might lie the origin of Sannyasa, the goal of human life is to become a knower of Brahman by embracing this vow of renunciation. The supreme end is to enter the life of Sannyasa. They alone are blessed indeed, who have broken off from worldly life through a spirit of renunciation. (VI. 509.)

13. If I do not find bliss in the life of the Spirit, shall I seek satisfaction in the life of the senses? If I cannot get nectar, shall I fall back upon ditch water? (V. 417.)

14. One may gain political and social independence, but if he is a slave to his passions and desires, he cannot feel the pure joy of real freedom. (V. 419.)

15. If a man throws aside the vanities of the world we hear him called mad, but such men are the salt of the earth. Out of such madness have come the powers that have moved this world of ours, and out of such madness alone will come the powers of the future that are going to move the world. (IV. 171.)

16. The real Sannyasin is a teacher of householders. It is with the light and teaching obtained from them that householders of old triumphed many a time in the battles of life. The householders give food and clothing to the Sadhus only in return for their invaluable teachings. Had there been no such mutual exchange in India, her people would have become extinct like the American Indians by this time. It is because the householders still give a few morsels of food to the Sadhus that they are yet able to keep their foothold on the path of progress. The Sannyasins are not idle. They are really the fountain-head of all activity. The householders see lofty ideals carried into practice in the lives of the Sadhus and accept from them such noble ideas; and this it is that has up till now enabled them to fight their battle of life from the sphere of Karma. The example of holy Sadhus makes them work out holy ideas in life and imbibe real energy for work. The Sannyasins inspire the householders in all noble causes by embodying in their lives the highest principle of giving up everything for the sake of God and the good of the world, and as a return the householders give them a few doles of food. And the very disposition and capacity to grow that food develops in the people because of the blessings and good wishes of the all-renouncing monks. It is because of their

failure to understand the deeper issues that people blame the monastic institution. Whatever may be the case in other countries, in this land the bark of householders' life does not sink only because the Sannyasins are at its helm. (VI. 510.)

17. With a view to certain ends we have to adopt certain means. These means vary according to the conditions of time, place, individual, etc., but the end always remains unaltered. In the case of the Sannyasin, the end is the liberation of the Self and doing good to humanity आत्मनो मोक्षार्थं जगद्धिताय च।—and of the ways to attain it, the renunciation of Kama-Kanchana is the most important. Remember, renunciation consists in the total absence of all selfish motives and not in mere abstinence from external contact, such as avoiding to touch one's money kept with another but at the same time enjoying all its benefits. Would that be renunciation? For accomplishing the two above-mentioned ends, the begging excursion would be a great help to a Sannyasin at a time when the householders strictly obeyed the injunctions of Manu and other law-givers, by setting apart every day a portion of their meal for ascetic guests. Nowadays things have changed considerably, especially in Bengal, where no Madhukari system prevails. Here it would be mere waste of energy to try to live on Madhukari, and you would profit

nothing by it. The injunction of Bhiksha (begging) is a means to serve the above two ends, which will not be served by that way now. It does not therefore go against the principle of renunciation under such circumstances if a Sannyasin provides for mere necessaries of life and devotes all his energy to the accomplishment of his ends for which he took Sannyasa. Attaching too much importance ignorantly to the means brings confusion. The end should never be lost sight of. (V. 261-62.)

18. In this country, (U.S.A.) the clergymen sometimes receive as high salaries as rupees thirty thousand, forty thousand, fifty thousand, even ninety thousand a year, for preaching two hours on Sunday only, and that only six months in a year. Look at the millions upon millions they spend for the support of their religion, and young Bengal has been taught that these Godlike, absolutely unselfish men like Kambli-Swami are idle vagabonds. मद्भक्तानां च ये भक्ता: ते मे भक्ततमा मता:—"Those who are devoted to My worshippers are regarded as the best of devotees."

Take even an extreme case, that of an extremely ignorant Vairagi. Even he, when he goes into a village, tries his best to impart to the villagers whatever he knows, from Tulsidas or *Chaitanya Charitamritam* or the Alwars in Southern India. Is that not doing some good?

And all this for only a bit of bread and a rag of cloth. Before unmercifully criticising them, think how much you do, my brother, for your poor fellow-countrymen, at whose expense you have got your education, and by grinding whose face you maintain your position and pay your teachers, for teaching you that the Babajis are only vagabonds. (IV. 339.)

19. The Sannyasin should have nothing to do with the rich, his duty is with the poor. He should treat the poor with loving care and serve them joyfully with all his might. To pay respects to the rich and hang on them for support has been the bane of all the Sannyasin communities of our country (India). A true Sannyasin should scrupulously avoid that. Such conduct becomes a public woman rather than one who professes to have renounced the world. (V. 260-61.)

20. A Sannyasin should avoid the food, bedding, etc., which have been touched or used by the householders, in order *to save himself*— not from hatred towards them—so long as he has not risen to the highest grade, that is, has not become a Paramahamsa. (VII. 410.)

21. To be *in* the world but not *of* it is the true test of the Sannyasin. (VIII. 9.)

22. Truth never comes where lust and fame and greed

SANNYASA OR THE MONASTIC LIFE

Of gain reside. No man who thinks of woman
As his wife can ever perfect be;
Nor he who owns the least of things, nor he
Whom anger chains, can ever pass thro' Maya's gates.
So, give these up, Sannyasin bold! Say—
"Om Tat Sat, Om!" (IV. 394.)

23. Where seekest thou? That freedom, friend, this world
Nor that can give. In books and temples vain
Thy search. Thine only is the hand that holds
The rope that drags thee on. Then cease lament,
Let go thy hold, Sannyasin bold; Say—
"Om Tat Sat, Om!" (IV. 394.)

24. Have thou no home. What home can hold thee, friend?
The sky thy roof, the grass thy bed, and food
What chance may bring; well cooked or ill, judge not.
No food or drink can taint that noble Self
Which knows Itself. Like rolling river free
Thou ever be, Sannyasin bold! Say—
"Om Tat Sat, Om!" (IV. 395.)

XL

SERVICE

1. From highest Brahman to the yonder
                                    worm,
   And to the very minutest atom,
   Everywhere is the same God, the
                                    All-Love;
   Friend, offer mind, soul, body, at their
                                    feet.
   These are His manifold forms before thee,
   Rejecting them, where seekest thou
                                    for God?
   Who loves all beings, without distinction,
   He indeed is worshipping best his God.
                                    (IV. 496.)

2. This is the gist of all worship—to be pure and to do good to others. He who sees Shiva in the poor, in the weak, and in the diseased, really worships Shiva; and if he sees Shiva only in the image, his worship is but preliminary. He who has served and helped one poor man seeing Shiva in him, without thinking of his caste, or creed, or race, or anything, with him Shiva is more pleased than with the man who sees Him only in temples. (III. 141.)

3. He who wants to serve the father must serve the children first. He who wants to serve

Shiva must serve His children—must serve all creatures in the world first. (III. 142.)

4. It is said in the Shastra that those who serve the servants of God are His greatest servants. So you will bear this in mind. (III. 142.)

5. Let me tell you again, that you must be pure and help anyone who comes to you as much as lies in your power. And this is good Karma. By the power of this, the heart becomes pure (Chitta Shuddhi), and then Shiva who is residing in every one, will become manifest. (III. 142.)

6. Selfishness is the chief sin, thinking of ourselves first. He who thinks "I will eat first, I will have more money than others, and I will possess everything"; he who thinks "I will get to heaven before others, I will get Mukti before others", is the selfish man. The unselfish man says, "I will be last, I do not care to go to heaven, I will go to hell, if by doing so I can help my brothers." This unselfishness is the test of religion. (III. 143.)

7. This life is short, the vanities of the world are transient, but they alone live who live for others, the rest are more dead than alive. (IV. 363.)

8. Do you love your fellow men? Where should you go to seek for God—are not all the poor, the miserable, the weak, gods? Why not

worship them first? Why go to dig a well on the shores of the Ganga? (V. 51.)

9. Who will give the world light? Sacrifice in the past has been the Law, it will be, alas, for ages to come. The earth's bravest and best will have to sacrifice themselves for the good of many, for the welfare of all. Buddhas by the hundred are necessary with eternal love and pity. (VII. 498.)

10. Religions of the world have become lifeless mockeries. What the world wants is character. The world is in need of those whose life is one burning love, selfless. That love will make every word tell like thunderbolt. (VII. 498.)

11. Awake, awake, great ones! The world is burning with misery. Can you sleep? Let us call and call till the sleeping gods awake, till the god within answers to the call. What more is in life? What greater work? (VII. 498.)

12. May I be born again and again, and suffer thousands of miseries so that I may worship the only God that exists, the only God I believe in, the sum total of all souls—and above all, my God the wicked, my God the miserable, my God the poor of all races, of all species, is the special object of my worship. (V. 137.)

13. Doing good to others out of compassion is good, but the Seva (service) of all beings in the spirit of the Lord is better. (V. 325.)

14. It is our privilege to be allowed to be charitable, for only so can we grow. The poor man suffers that we may be helped; let the giver kneel down and give thanks, let the receiver stand up and permit. See the Lord back of every being and give to Him. (VII. 68.)

15. Doing work is not religion, but work done rightly leads to Freedom. In reality all pity is darkness, because whom to pity? Can you pity God? And is there anything else? Thank God for giving you this world as a moral gymnasium to help your development, but never imagine you can help the world. (VII. 69.)

16. Self-sacrifice, not self-assertion, is the highest law of the universe.... Religion comes with intense self-sacrifice. Desire nothing for yourself. Do all for others. This is to live and move and have your being in God. (VI. 83.)

17. Selfishness is the devil incarnate in every man. Every bit of self, bit by bit, is devil. Take off self by one side and God enters by the other. (VI. 119.)

18. The highest ideal is eternal and entire self-abnegation, where there is no "I" but all is "thou". (I. 84-85.)

19. Unselfishness is God. (I. 87.)

20. Are you unselfish? That is the question. If you are, you will be perfect without reading a

single religious book, without going into a single church or temple. (I. 93.)

21. The difference between God and the devil is in nothing except in unselfishness and selfishness. (I. 425.)

22. It is a privilege to serve mankind, for this is the worship of God; God is here, in all these human souls. He is the soul of man. (I. 424.)

23. Be grateful to the man you help, think of him as God. Is it not a great privilege to be allowed to worship God by helping your fellow men? (I. 77.)

24. The world is a grand moral gymnasium wherein we have all to take exercise so as to become stronger and stronger spiritually. (I. 80.)

25. The first of everything should go to the poor; we have only a right to what remains. The poor are God's representatives; any one that suffers is His representative. (IV. 10.)

XLI

STRENGTH

1. This is a great fact: strength is life; weakness is death. Strength is felicity, life eternal, immortal; weakness is constant strain and misery: weakness is death. (II. 3.)

2. Men are taught from childhood that they are weak and sinners. Teach them that they are all glorious children of immortality, even those who are the weakest in manifestation. Let positive, strong, helpful thought enter into their brains from very childhood. Lay yourself open to these thoughts, and not to weakening and paralysing ones. Say to your own minds, "I am He, I am He". Let it ring day and night in your minds like a song, and at the point of death declare: "I am He". That is truth; the infinite strength of the world is yours. (II. 87.)

3. As soon as you say, "I am bound", "I am weak", "I am helpless", woe unto you; you rivet one more chain upon yourself. Do not say it, do not think it. (II. 198.)

4. It is weakness, says the Vedanta, which is the cause of all misery in this world. Weakness is the one cause of suffering. We become miserable because we are weak. We lie, steal, kill and commit other crimes, because we are

weak. We die because we are weak. Where there is nothing to weaken us, there is no death nor sorrow. We are miserable through delusion. Give up the delusion and the whole thing vanishes. (II. 198.)

5. This is the one question I put to every man, woman or child, when they are in physical, mental or spiritual training: Are you strong? Do you feel strength?—for I know it is truth alone that gives strength. I know that truth alone gives life, and nothing but going towards reality will make us strong, and none will reach truth until he is strong. Every system, therefore, which weakens the mind, makes one superstitious, makes one mope, makes one desire all sorts of wild impossibilities, mysteries and superstitions, I do not like, because its effect is dangerous. Such systems never bring any good; such things create morbidity in the mind, make it weak, so weak that in course of time it will be almost impossible to receive truth or live up to it. Strength, therefore, is the one thing needful. (II. 201.)

6. I am responsible for my fate, I am the bringer of good unto myself, I am the bringer of evil. I am the Pure and Blessed One. We must reject all thoughts that assert to the contrary. (II. 202.)

7. This is the only way to reach the goal, to

tell ourselves, and to tell everybody else, that we are divine. And as we go on repeating this, strength comes. He who falters at first will get stronger and stronger, and the voice will increase in volume until the truth takes possession of our hearts, and courses through our veins, and permeates our bodies. (II. 202.)

8. Those that blame others—and, alas! the number of them is increasing every day—are generally miserable, with helpless brains; they have brought themselves to that pass through their own mistakes and blame others, but this does not alter their position. It does not serve them in any way. This attempt to throw the blame upon others only weakens them the more. Therefore, blame none for your own faults, stand upon your own feet, and take the whole responsibility upon yourselves. Say, "This misery that I am suffering is of my own doing, and that very thing proves that it will have to be undone by me alone." That which I created, I can demolish; that which is created by some one else I shall never be able to destroy. Therefore, stand up, be bold, be strong. (II. 225.)

9. All the strength and succour you want is within yourselves. Therefore, make your own future. "Let the dead past bury its dead." The infinite future is before you, and you must always remember that each word, thought and deed,

lays up a store for you and that as the bad thoughts and bad works are ready to spring upon you like tigers, so also there is the inspiring hope that the good thoughts, and good deeds, are ready with the power of a hundred thousand angels to defend you always and for ever. (II. 225.)

10. The remedy for weakness is not brooding over weakness, but thinking of strength that is already within them. Instead of telling them they are sinners, the Vedanta takes the opposite position, and says, "You are pure and perfect, and what you call sin does not belong to you". Sins are low degrees of Self-manifestation; manifest your Self in a high degree. That is the one thing to remember; all of us can do that. Never say, "No"; never say, "I cannot", for you are infinite. Even time and space are as nothing compared with your nature. You can do anything and everything, you are almighty. (II. 300.)

11. What makes a man stand up and work? Strength. Strength is goodness, weakness is sin. If there is one word that you find coming out like a bomb from the Upanishads, bursting like a bomb-shell upon masses of ignorance: it is the word, fearlessness. And the only religion that ought to be taught, is the religion of *fearlessness*. Either in this world or in the world of religion, it is true that fear is the sure cause of degrada-

tion and sin. It is fear that brings misery, fear that brings death, fear that breeds evil. And what causes fear? Ignorance of our own nature. (III. 160.)

12. Take off the veil of hypnotism which you have cast upon the world, send not out thoughts and words of weakness unto humanity. Know that all sins and all evils can be summed up in that one word, weakness. It is weakness that is the motive power in all evil doing; it is weakness that makes men injure others; it is weakness that makes them manifest what they are not in reality. Let them know what they really are; let them repeat day and night what they are.... Let them suck it in with their mother's milk, this idea of strength—I am He, I am He. (III. 426.)

13. Infinite strength is religion and God. Avoid weakness and slavery. (VII. 13.)

14. Strength, strength for us. What we need is strength, who will give us strength? There are thousands to weaken us, and of stories we have had enough.... Everything that can weaken us as a race we have had for the last thousand years. It seeems as if during that period the national life had this one end in view, viz how to make us weaker and weaker, till we have become real earthworms, crawling at the feet of every one who dares to put his foot on us. Therefore, my friends, as one of your blood, as one that lives

and dies with you, let me tell you that we want strength, strength, and every time strength. (III. 238.)

15. The best guide in life is strength. In religion, as in all other matters, discard everything that weakens you, have nothing to do with it. (I. 134.)

XLII

UPANISHADS

1. The Jnanakanda of the Vedas comprises the Upanishads and is known by the name of Vedanta, the pinnacle of the Shrutis, as it is called. Wherever you find the Âchâryas quoting a passage from the Shrutis, it is invariably from the Upanishads. The Vedanta is now the religion of the Hindus. If any sect in India wants to have its ideas established with a firm hold on the people, it must base them on the authority of the Vedanta. (III. 456.)

2. All the books contained in the Upanishads have one subject, one task before them—to prove the following theme: "Just as by the knowledge of one lump of clay we have the knowledge of all the clay in the universe, so what is that, knowing which we know everything in the universe?" (I. 362.)

3. The Upanishads are the great mine of strength. Therein lies strength enough to invigorate the whole world; the whole world can be vivified, made strong, energised through them. They will call with trumpet voice upon the weak, the miserable and the downtrodden of all races, all creeds and all sects, to stand on their feet and be free; freedom, physical freedom, mental free-

dom and spiritual freedom are the watchword of the Upanishads. (III. 238.)

4. In modern language, the theme of the Upanishads is to find an ultimate unity of things. Knowledge is nothing but finding unity in the midst of diversity. Every science is based upon this; all human knowledge is based upon the finding of unity in the midst of diversity, and if it is the task of small fragments of human knowledge, which we call our sciences, to find unity in the midst of a few different phenomena, the task becomes stupendous when the theme before us is to find unity in the midst of this marvellously diversified universe, where prevail unnumbered differences in name and form, in matter and spirit—each thought differing from every other thought, each form differing from every other form. Yet, to harmonise these many planes and unending Lokas, in the midst of this infinite variety to find unity, is the theme of the Upanishads. (III. 397-98.)

5. In the Upanishads, we see a tremendous departure made. It is declared that these heavens, in which men live with the ancestors after death, cannot be permanent, seeing that everything which has name and form must die. If there are heavens with forms, these heavens must vanish in course of time; they may last millions of years, but there must come a time

when they will have to go. With this idea came another, that these souls must come back to earth, and that heavens are places where they enjoy the results of their good works, and after these effects are finished they come back into this earth life again. (II. 316-17.)

6. I want to bring to your notice one or two points in the study of the Upanishads. In the first place, they are the most wonderful poems in the world. If you read the Samhita portion of the Vedas, you now and then find passages of most marvellous beauty. For instance, the famous Shloka which describes Chaos—तम आसीत् तमसा गूढमग्रे etc., "When darkness was hidden in darkness", so on it goes. One reads and feels the wonderful sublimity of the poetry. Do you mark this, that outside of India, and inside also, there have been attempts at painting the sublime. But outside, it has always been the infinite in the muscles, the external world, the infinite of matter, or of space. When Milton or Dante, or any other great European poet, either ancient or modern, wants to paint a picture of the Infinite, he tries to soar outside, to make you feel the Infinite through the muscles. That attempt has been made here also. You find it in the Samhitas, the Infinite of extension, most marvellously painted and placed before the

readers, such as has been done, nowhere else. (III. 329-30.)

7. Just as the Greek mind, or the modern European mind wants to find the solution of life and of all the sacred problems of Being by searching into the external world, so also did our forefathers, and just as the Europeans failed, they failed also. But the Western people never made a move more, they remained there, they failed in the search for the solution of the great problems of life and death in the external world, and there they remained, stranded; our forefathers also found it impossible, but were bolder in declaring the utter helplessness of the senses to find the solution. Nowhere else was the answer better put than in the Upanishad! यतो वाचो निवर्तन्ते अप्राप्य मनसा सह। "From whence the word comes back reflected, together with the mind." न तत्र चक्षुर्गच्छति न वाग्गच्छति। "There the eye cannot go, nor can speech reach." There are various sentences which declare the utter helplessness of the senses, but they do not stop there; they fell back upon the internal nature of man, they went to get the answer from their own soul, they became introspective; they gave up external nature as a failure, as nothing could be done there, as no hope, no answer, could be found; they discovered the dull, dead matter would not

give them truth, and they fell back upon the shining soul of man, and there, the answer was found. (III. 330-31.)

8. The one central idea throughout all the Upanishads is that of realisation. (II. 170.)

9. तमेवैकं जानथ आत्मानम् अन्या वाचो विमुञ्चथ —"Know this Atman alone", they declared, "give up all other vain words, and hear no other." In the Atman they found the solution—the greatest of all Atmans, the God, the Lord of this Universe, His relation to the Atman of man, our duty to Him, and through that our relation to each other. And herein you find the most sublime poetry in the world. No more is the attempt made to paint this Atman in the language of matter. Nay, for it they have given up even all positive language. No more is there any attempt to come to the senses to give them the idea of the Infinite, no more is there an external, dull, dead, material, spacious, sensuous infinite, but instead of that comes something, which is as fine as even that mentioned in the saying:

न तत्र सूर्यो भाति न चन्द्रतारकं
नेमा विद्युतो भान्ति कुतोऽयमग्निः ।
तमेव भान्तमनुभाति सर्वं
तस्य भासा सर्वमिदं विभाति ॥

—"There the sun cannot illumine, nor the moon,

nor the stars, there this flash of lightning cannot illumine; what to speak of this mortal fire!" What poetry in the world can be more sublime than this! Such poetry you find nowhere else. (III. 331.)

10. We now come to the teachings of the Upanishads. Various texts are there. Some are Monistic. But there are certain doctrines which are agreed to by all the different sects of India. First, there is the doctrine of Samsara, or reincarnation of the soul. Secondly, they all agree in their psychology; first there is the body, behind that, what they call the Sukshma-Sharira, the mind, and behind that even, is the Jiva. That is the great difference between Western and Indian Psychology; in the Western Psychology the mind is the soul, here it is not. The Antah-karana, the internal instrument, as the mind is called, is only an instrument in the hands of Jiva, through which the Jiva works on the body, or on the external world. Here they all agree, and they all also agree that this Jiva, or Atman, Jivatman as it is called by various sects, is eternal, without beginning; and that it is going from birth to birth, until it gets a final release. They all agree in this, and they also all agree in one other most vital point, which alone marks characteristically, most prominently, most vitally, the difference between the Indian and the

Western mind, and it is this, that everything is in the soul. There is no inspiration, but properly speaking, expiration. All powers and all purity and all greatness—everything is in the soul. (III. 334.)

11. Thus it is that the Vedas proclaim not a dreadful combination of unforgiving laws, not an endless prison of cause and effect, but that at the head of all these laws, in and through every particle of matter and force, stands One, "By whose command the wind blows, the fire burns, the clouds rain, and death stalks upon the earth." (I. 11.)

XLIII

VEDANTA: ITS THEORY AND PRACTICE

1. Materialism says, the voice of freedom is a delusion. Idealism says, the voice that tells of bondage is delusion. Vedanta says, you are free and not free at the same time; never free on the earthly plane, but ever free on the spiritual. (VII. 32.)

2. This philosophy is very, very ancient; it is the outcome of that mass of ancient Aryan literature known by the name of the Vedas. It is, as it were, the very flower of all the speculations and experiences and analyses, embodied in that mass of literature—collected and culled through centuries. This Vedanta philosophy has certain peculiarities. In the first place, it is perfectly impersonal; it does not owe its origin to any person or prophet; it does not build itself around one man as a centre. Yet it has nothing to say against philosophies, which do build themselves around certain persons. (I. 387-88.)

3. The Vedanta Philosophy, as it is generally called at the present day, really comprises all the various sects that now exist in India. Thus there have been various interpretations, and to my mind they have been progressive, beginning with

the Dualistic or Dvaita and ending with the non-dualistic or Advaita. (I. 357.)

4. Vedanta and modern science both posit a self-evolving Cause. In Itself are all the causes. Take for example, the potter shaping a pot. The potter is the primal cause, the clay the material cause, and the wheel the instrumental cause; but the Atman is all three. Atman is cause and manifestation too. The Vedantist says, the universe is not real, it is only apparent. Nature is God seen through nescience. The Pantheists say, God has become nature or this world; the Advaitists affirm that God is appearing as this world, but He is not this world. (VII. 50.)

5. The Vedanta claims that man is divine, that all this which we see around us is the outcome of that consciousness of the divine. Everything that is strong, and good and powerful in human nature is the outcome of that divinity, and though potential in many, there is no difference between man and man essentially, all being alike divine. There is, as it were, an infinite ocean behind, and you and I are so many waves, coming out of that infinite ocean; and each one of us is trying our best to manifest that infinite outside. (I. 388.)

6. Another peculiar idea of the Vedanta is that we must allow this infinite variation in religious thought, and not try to bring everybody

to the same opinion, because the goal is the same; as the Vedantist says in his poetical language:

"As so many rivers, having their source in different mountains, roll down, crooked or straight, and at last come into the ocean—so, all these various creeds and religions, taking their start from different standpoints and running through crooked or straight courses, at last come into Thee." (I. 390.)

7. Vedanta does not take the position that this world is only a miserable one. That would be untrue. At the same time, it is a mistake to say that this world is full of happiness and blessings. So it is useless to tell children that this world is all good, all flowers, and milk and honey. That is what we have all dreamt. At the same time it is erroneous to think, because one man has suffered more than another, that all is evil. It is this duality, this play of good and evil that makes our world of experiences. At the same time the Vedanta says, "Do not think that good and evil are two, are two separate essences, for they are one and the same thing appearing in different degrees and in different guises and producing differences of feeling in the same mind." (II. 179-80.)

8. The Vedanta system begins with tremendous pessimism, and ends with real optimism. We deny the sense optimism but assert the real

optimism of the Supersensuous. That real happiness is not in the senses but above the senses; and it is in every man. The sort of optimism which we see in the world is what will lead to ruin through the senses. (V. 283.)

9. The theme of the Vedanta is to see the Lord in everything, to see things in their real nature, not as they appear to be. (II. 312.)

10. The Vedanta says that you are pure and perfect, and that there is a state beyond good and evil, and that is your own nature. It is higher than good. Good is only a lesser differentiation than evil.

We have no theory of evil. We call it ignorance. (V. 282.)

11. Vedanta declares that religion is here and now, because the question of this life and that life, of life and death, this world and that world, is merely one of superstition and prejudice. There is no break in time beyond what we make. What difference is there between ten and twelve o'clock except what we make by certain changes in nature? Time flows on the same. So what is meant by this life or that life? It is only a question of time, and what is lost in time may be made up by speed in work. So, says the Vedanta, religion is to be realised now. And for you to become religious means that you will start without any religion, work your way up and realise

things, see things for yourself; and when you have done that, then, and then alone, you have religion. Before that you are no better than atheists, or worse, because the atheist is sincere; he stands up and says, "I do not know about these things", while those others do not know but go about the world saying, "We are very religious people." (VI. 13.)

12. Materialism prevails in Europe today. You may pray for the salvation of the modern sceptics, but they do not yield, they want reason. The salvation of Europe depends on a rationalistic religion, and Advaita—the non-duality, the Oneness, the idea of the impersonal God—is the only religion that can have any hold on any intellectual people. It comes whenever religion seems to disappear, and irreligion seems to prevail, and that is why it has taken ground in Europe and America. (II. 139.)

13. I make bold to say that the only religion which agrees with, and even goes a little further than modern researches, both on physical and moral lines, is the Advaita, and that is why it appeals to modern scientists so much. They find that the old dualistic theories are not enough for them, do not satisfy their necessities. (II. 138.)

14. Another peculiarity of the Advaita system is that from its very start it is non-destructive. This is another glory, the boldness to preach;

"Do not disturb the faith of any, even of those who through ignorance have attached themselves to lower forms of woship." That is what it says, do not disturb, but help everyone to get higher and higher; include all humanity. (II. 141.)

15. The Dualists all the world over naturally believe in a Personal God who is purely anthropomorphic, who like a great potentate in this world, is pleased with some and displeased with others. He is arbitrarily pleased with some people or races and showers blessing upon them. Naturally the Dualist comes to the conclusion that God has favourites, and he hopes to be one of them. You will find that in almost every religion is the idea, "We are the favourites of our God, and only by believing as we do, can you be taken into favour with Him." Some Dualists are so narrow as to insist that only the few that have been predestined to the favour of God can be saved; the rest may try ever so hard, but they cannot be accepted. I challenge you to show me one Dualistic religion which has not more or less of this exclusiveness. And, therefore, in the nature of things Dualistic religions are bound to fight and quarrel with each other, and this they have ever been doing. (II. 142.)

16. This idea of reincarnation runs parallel with the other doctrine of the eternity of the human soul. Nothing which ends at one point

can be without a beginning and nothing that begins at one point can be without an end. We cannot believe in such a monstrous impossibility as the beginning of the human soul. The doctrine of reincarnation asserts the freedom of the soul. (I. 319-20.)

17. Those that come out of zero will certainly have to go back to zero. Neither you, nor I, nor anyone present, has come out of zero, nor will go back to zero. We have been existing eternally, and will exist, and there is no power under the sun, or above the sun, which can undo your or my existence, or send us back to zero. Now this idea of reincarnation is not only not a frightening idea, but is most essential for the moral well-being of the human race. It is the only logical conclusion that thoughtful men can arrive at. If you are going to exist in eternity hereafter, it must be that you have existed through eternity in the past: it cannot be otherwise. (II. 217-18.)

18. The Atman never comes nor goes, is never born nor dies. It is nature moving before the Atman, and the reflection of this motion is on the Atman and the Atman ignorantly thinks it is moving, and not nature. When the Atman thinks that, it is bondage, but when it comes to find it never moves, that it is omnipresent, then freedom comes. The Atman in bondage is called Jiva.

Thus you see that when it is said that the Atman comes and goes, it is said only for facility of understanding, just as for convenience, in studying astronomy you are asked to suppose that the sun moves round the earth, though such is not the case. So the Jiva, the soul, comes to higher or lower states. This is the well-known law of reincarnation, and this law binds all creation. (II. 257-58.)

19. The aim and end in this life for the Jnana-Yogi is to become this Jivanmukta, "living-free". He is Jivanmukta who can live in this world without being attached. He is like the lotus leaves in water, which are never wetted by the water. He is the highest of human beings, nay, the highest of all beings, for he has realised his identity with the Absolute, he has realised that he is one with God. (III. 10-11.)

20. So, what is left attached to the man who has reached the Self and seen the truth, is the remnant of the good impressions of past life, the good momentum. Even if he lives in the body and works incessantly, he works only to do good; his lips speak only benediction to all; his hands do only good works; his mind can only think good thoughts; his presence is a blessing wherever he goes. (II. 284.)

21. There are some who do not understand Advaitism and make a travesty of its teachings.

They say, what is Shuddha and Ashuddha, what is the difference between virtue and vice—it is all human superstitions—and observe no normal restraint in their actions. It is downright roguery, and any amount of harm is done by the preaching of such things.

This body is made up of two sorts of Karma consisting of virtue and vice—injurious vice and non-injurious virtue. A thorn is pricking my body, and I take another thorn to take it out and then throw both away. A man desiring to be perfect takes a thorn of virtue and with it takes off the thorn of vice. He still lives, and virtue alone being left, the momentum of action left to him must be of virtue. A bit of holiness is left to the Jivanmukta and he lives, but everything he does must be holy. (VI. 111.)

22. If I teach you, therefore, that your nature is evil, that you should go home and sit in sackcloth and ashes and weep your lives out because you took certain false steps, it will not help you, but will weaken you all the more, and I shall be showing you the road to more evil than good. If this room is full of darkness for thousands of years and you come in and begin to weep and wail, "Oh the darkness", will the darkness vanish? Strike a match and light comes in a moment. What good will it do you to think all your lives, "Oh, I have done evil, I have made

many mistakes"? It requires no ghost to tell us that. Bring in the light and the evil goes in a moment. Build up your character, and manifest your real nature, the Effulgent, the Resplendent, the Ever-Pure, and call It up in everyone that you see. I wish that everyone of us had come to such a state that even in the vilest of human beings we could see the Real Self within, and instead of condemning them, say, "Rise thou effulgent one, rise thou who art always pure, rise thou birthless and deathless, rise almighty, and manifest thy true nature. These little manifestations do not befit thee." This is the highest prayer that the Advaita teaches. This is the one prayer, to remember our true nature, the God who is always within us, thinking of it always as infinite, almighty, ever-good, ever-beneficent, selfless, bereft of all limitations. And because that nature is selfless, it is strong and fearless; for only to selfishness comes fear. He who has nothing to desire for himself, whom does he fear, and what can frighten him? What fear has death for him? What fear has evil for him? So if we are Advaitists, we must think from this moment that our old self is dead and gone. The old Mr., Mrs., and Miss So-and-so are gone, they were mere superstitions, and what remains is the ever-pure, the ever-strong, the almighty, the all-knowing— that alone remains for us, and then all fear vanishes from us. Who can injure us, the omnipresent? All weakness has vanished from us, and our only work is to arouse this knowledge in our fellow-beings. We see that they too are the same pure self, only they do not know it; we must teach them, we must help them to rouse up their infinite nature. This is what I feel to be absolutely necessary all over the world. These doctrines are old, older than many mountains possibly. All truth is eternal. Truth is nobody's property; no race, no individual can lay any exclusive claim to it. Truth is the nature of all souls. Who can lay any special claim to it? But it has to be made practical, to be made simple (for the highest truths are always simple), so that it may penetrate every pore of human society, and become the property of the highest intellects and the commonest minds, of the man, woman, and child at the same time. All these ratiocinations of logic, all these bundles of metaphysics, all these theologies and ceremonies may have been good in their own time, but let us try to make things simpler and bring about the golden days when every man will be a worshipper, and the Reality in every man will be the object of worship. (II. 357-58.)

23. The Vedanta says that not only can this be realised in the depths of forests or caves, but by men in all possible conditions of life. We

have seen that the people who discovered these truths were neither living in caves nor forests, nor following the ordinary vocations of life, but men who, we have every reason to believe, led the busiest of lives, men who had to command armies, to sit on thrones, and look to the welfare of millions—and all these, in the days of absolute monarchy, and not as in these days when a king is to a great extent a mere figure-head. Yet they could find time to think out all these thoughts, to realise them, and to teach them to humanity. How much more then should it be practical for us whose lives, compared with theirs, are lives of leisure? That we cannot realise them is a shame to us, seeing that we are comparatively free all the time, having very little to do. My requirements are as nothing compared with those of an ancient absolute monarch. My wants are as nothing compared with the demands of Arjuna on the battlefield of Kurukshetra, commanding a huge army; and yet he could find time in the midst of the din and turmoil of battle to talk the highest philosophy and to carry it into his life also. Surely we ought to be able to do as much in this life of ours—comparatively free, easy, and comfortable. Most of us here have more time than we think we have, if we really want to use it for good. With the amount of freedom we have we can attain to two hundred ideals in this life, if we will, but we must not degrade the ideal to the actual. One of the most insinuating things comes to us in the shape of persons who apologise for our mistakes and teach us how to make special excuses for all our foolish wants and foolish desires; and we think that their ideal is the only ideal we need have. But it is not so. The Vedanta teaches no such thing. The actual should be reconciled to the ideal, the present life should be made to coincide with life eternal. (II. 296-97.)

24. We want to worship a living God. I have seen nothing but God all my life, nor have you. To see this chair you first see God, and then the chair in and through Him. He is everywhere saying, "I am." The moment you feel "I am", you are conscious of Existence. Where shall we go to find God if we cannot see Him in our own hearts and in every living being? "Thou art the man, Thou art the woman. Thou art the girl, and Thou art the boy. Thou art the old man tottering with a stick. Thou art the young man walking in the pride of strength." Thou art all that exists, a wonderful living God who is the only fact in the universe. This seems to many to be a terrible contradiction to the traditional God who lives behind a veil somewhere and whom nobody ever sees. The priests only give us an assurance that if we follow them, listen to their admoni-

tions, and walk in the way they mark out for us—then when we die, they will give us a passport to enable us to see the face of God! What are all these heaven ideas but simply modifications of this nonsensical priestcraft?

Of course the Impersonal idea is very destructive; it takes away all trade from the priests, churches, and temples. In India there is a famine now, but there are temples in each one of which there are jewels worth a king's ransom! If the priests taught this Impersonal idea to the people, their occupation would be gone. Yet we have to teach it unselfishly, without priestcraft. You are God and so am I; who obeys whom? Who worships whom? You are the highest temple of God; I would rather worship you than any temple, image, or Bible....But what is more practical than worshipping here, worshipping you? I see you, feel you, and I know you are God. The Mohammedan says, there is no God but Allah. The Vedanta says, there is nothing that is not God. (II. 320-21.)

25. Vedanta teaches the God that is in everyone, has become everyone and everything.... The kingdom of heaven went from Vedanta hundreds of years ago. Vedanta is concerned only with spirituality.... God is spirit and He should be worshipped in spirit and in truth. (VIII. 125-26.)

26. These are what Vedanta has not to give. No book. No man to be singled out from the rest of mankind—"You are worms, and we are the Lord God!"—none of that. If you are the Lord God, I also am the Lord God. So Vedanta knows no sin. There are mistakes but no sin; and in the long run everything is going to be all right. No Satan—none of this nonsense. Vedanta believes in only one sin, only one in the world, and it is this: the moment you think you are a sinner or anybody is a sinner, that is sin. From that follows every other mistake or what is usually called sin. There have been many mistakes in our lives. But we are going on. Glory be unto us that we have made mistakes! Take a long look at your past life. If your present condition is good, it has been caused by all the past mistakes as well as successes. Glory be unto success! Glory be unto mistakes! ...

You see, Vedanta proposes no sin nor sinner. No God to be afraid of. He is the one being of whom we shall never be afraid, because He is our own Self. There is only one being of whom you cannot possibly be afraid; He is that. Then isn't it really the most superstitious person who has fear of God? There may be someone who is afraid of his shadow; but even he is not afraid of himself. God is man's very Self. He is the one being whom you can never possibly fear. What is all this nonsense, the fear of the Lord entering into a man, making him tremble and so on? Lord bless us that we are not all in the lunatic asylum! But if most of us are not lunatics, why should we invent such ideas as fear of God? Lord Buddha said that the whole human race is lunatic, more or less. It is perfectly true, it seems.

No book, no person, no Personal God. All these must go. Again, the senses must go. We cannot be bound to the senses. At present we are tied down—like persons dying of cold in the glaciers. They feel such a strong desire to sleep, and when their friends try to wake them, warning them of death, they say, "Let me die, I want to sleep". We all cling to the little things of the senses, even if we are ruined thereby; we forget there are much greater things. (VIII. 126-27.)

27. What does Vedanta teach us? In the first place, it teaches that you need not even go out of yourself to know the truth. All the past and all the future are here in the present. No man ever saw the past. Did any one of you see the past? When you think you are knowing the past, you only imagine the past in the present moment. To see the future, you would have to bring it down to the present, which is the only reality—the rest is imagination. This present is all that is. There is only the One.

All is here right now. One moment in infinite time is quite as complete and all-inclusive as every other moment. All that is and was and will be is here in the present. Let anybody try to imagine anything outside of it—he will not succeed. (VIII. 128.)

28. Therefore the Vedanta formulates, not a universal brotherhood, but universal oneness. I am the same as any other man, as any other animal—good, bad, anything. It is one body, one mind, one soul throughout. Spirit never dies. There is no death anywhere, not even for the body. Not even the mind dies. How can even the body die? One leaf may fall—does the tree die? The universe is my body. See how it continues. All minds are mine. With all feet I walk. Through all mouths I speak. In everybody I reside. (VIII. 129.)

XLIV

YOGA

1. Each soul is potentially divine.

The goal is to manifest this divinity within, by controlling nature, external and internal.

Do this either by work, or worship, or psychic control, or philosophy—by one, or more, or all of these—and be free.

This is the whole of religion. Doctrines, or dogmas, or rituals, or books, or temples, or forms, are but secondary details. (I. 257.)

2. The ultimate goal of all mankind, the aim and end of all religions, is but one—re-union with God, or, what amounts to the same, with the divinity which is every man's true nature. But while the aim is one, the method of attaining may vary with the different temperaments of men. Both the goal and the methods employed for reaching it are called Yoga, a word derived from the same Sanskrit root as the English "yoke", meaning "to join", to join us to our reality, God. There are various such Yogas, or methods of union—but the chief ones are Karma-Yoga, Bhakti-Yoga, Raja-Yoga, and Jnana-Yoga. (V. 291-92.)

3. As every science has its methods, so has every religion. The methods of attaining the end

of religion are called Yoga by us, and the different forms of Yoga that we teach, are adapted to the different natures and temperaments of men. We classify them in the following way, under four heads:

(1) Karma-Yoga—The manner in which a man realises his own divinity through works and duty.
(2) Bhakti-Yoga—The realisation of the divinity through devotion to, and love of, a Personal God.
(3) Raja-Yoga—The realisation of the divinity through the control of mind.
(4) Jnana-Yoga—The realisation of a man's own divinity through knowledge.

These are all different roads leading to the same centre—God. (V. 292.)

4. Each one of our Yogas is fitted to make man perfect even without the help of the others, because they have all the same goal in view. The Yogas of work, of wisdom, and of devotion are all capable of serving as direct and independent means for the attainment of Moksha. (I. 93.)

5. Non-attachment is the basis of all the Yogas. The man who gives up living in houses, wearing fine clothes, and eating good food, and goes into the desert, may be a most attached person. His only possession, his own body, may become everything to him; and as he lives he will be

simply struggling for the sake of his body. (I. 101.)

6. Vairagya or renunciation is the turning point in all the various Yogas. The Karmi (worker) renounces the fruits of his work. The Bhakta (devotee) renounces all little loves for the almighty and omnipresent love. The Yogi renounces his experiences, because his philosophy is that the whole Nature, although it is for the experience of the soul, at last brings him to know that he is not in Nature, but eternally separate from Nature. The Jnani (philosopher) renounces everything, because his philosophy is that Nature never existed, neither in the past, nor present, nor will be in the future. (III. 19.)

7. We claim that concentrating the powers of the mind is the only way to knowledge. In external science, concentration of mind is—putting it on something external; and in internal science, it is—drawing towards one's self. We call this concentration of mind, Yoga.

The Yogis claim a good deal. They claim that by concentration of the mind every truth in the universe becomes evident to the mind, both external and internal truth. (V. 299.)

8. The Yogis claim that of all the energies that are in the human body the highest is what they call "Ojas". Now this Ojas is stored up in the brain, and the more Ojas is in a man's head,

the more powerful he is, the more intellectual, the more spiritually strong. One man may speak beautiful language and beautiful thought, but they do not impress people; another man speaks neither beautiful language nor beautiful thoughts, yet his words charm. Every movement of his is powerful. That is the power of Ojas. (I. 169.)

9. All the forces that are working in the body in their highest become Ojas. You must remember that it is only a question of transformation. The same force which is working outside as electricity or magnetism, will become changed into inner force; the same forces that are working as muscular energy will be changed into Ojas. The Yogis say that that part of the human energy which is expressed as sex energy, in sexual thought, when checked and controlled, easily becomes changed into Ojas, and as the Muladhara guides these, the Yogi pays particular attention to that centre. He tries to take all this sexual energy and convert it into Ojas. It is only the chaste man or woman who can make the Ojas rise and store it in the brain; that is why chastity has always been considered the highest virtue. A man feels that if he is unchaste, spirituality goes away, he loses mental vigour and moral stamina. That is why in all the religious orders in the world which have produced spirit-

ual giants you will always find absolute chastity insisted upon. That is why the monks came into existence, giving up marriage. There must be perfect chastity in thought, word and deed; without it the practice of Raja-Yoga is dangerous, and may lead to insanity. (I. 170.)

10. The utility of this science is to bring out the perfect man, and not let him wait and wait for ages, just a plaything in the hands of the physical world, like a log of drift-wood carried from wave to wave, and tossing about in the ocean. This science wants you to be strong, to take the work in your own hand, instead of leaving it in the hands of Nature, and get beyond this little life. That is the great idea. (II. 19.)

11. Anything that is secret and mysterious in these systems of Yoga should be at once rejected. The best guide in life is strength. In religion, as in all other matters, discard everything that weakens you, have nothing to do with it. Mystery-mongering weakens the human brain. It has well-nigh destroyed Yoga—one of the greatest of sciences. (I. 134.)

12. He is indeed a Yogi who sees himself in the whole universe and the whole universe in himself. (VI. 83.)

13. This is no child's play, no fad to be tried one day and discarded the next. It is a life's

work; and the end to be attained is well worth all that it can cost us to reach it, being nothing less than the realisation of our absolute oneness with the Divine. (V. 294.)